PORN IS
"MENTAL"

Mental health crises caused by PORN consumption

WAEL IBRAHIM

First published by Ultimate World Publishing 2023
Copyright © 2023 Wael Ibrahim

ISBN

Paperback - 978-1-922982-38-4
Ebook - 978-1-922982-39-1

Cover design: Muhammad Ehtesham
Layout and typesetting: Ultimate World Publishing
Editor: Marinda Wilkinson

Ultimate World Publishing
Diamond Creek,
Victoria Australia 3089
www.writeabook.com.au

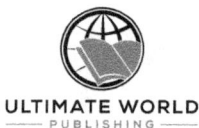

PRAISE FOR
PORN IS MENTAL

Through *Porn is Mental* you will gain a deeper understanding of the root causes of porn addiction. The author also must be commended for the strong focus on highlighting the multifaceted damage caused by porn. What further sets this book apart is its emphasis on the importance of seeking support and assistance in overcoming addiction. Wael Ibrahim recognises that addiction is a complex and challenging issue, and he encourages help to be sought from a trusted friend, family member, or professional.

Overall, *Porn is Mental* offers hope and healing to anyone who is struggling with addiction to pornography. It is a must-read for those looking to better understand the impact of porn on mental health and those seeking guidance on how to overcome this addiction.

~ Dr Zuleyha Keskin, Associate Head of School, Centre for Islamic Studies, Charles Sturt University

Porn is Mental is a comprehensive compilation which summaries all of the possibly known mental conditions caused or aggravated by porn use and addiction; and vice versa. In ways it seems encyclopedic, and we see it offering value to trained psychologists and sex therapists in identifying the most probable mental conditions afflicting the porn addicts in their care, with suggestions for management and response strategies to assist in devising a targeted intervention strategy. The real-life anecdotes found in some chapters would be of great help to concerned friends or relatives in recognising early warning signs of addiction in their loved ones, allowing them to offer well-informed advice and support towards treatment and healing. The learning objectives opening each chapter, coupled with heavily footnoted references of academic research and studies give students of porn-addiction treatment a solid basis to further their understanding of the subject. We share Wael's hope that porn use is not belittled as a harmless source of recreation but is recognised as the very serious epidemic that it already is.

~ Enon Mansor and Osman Sidek, authors of *Sex, Soul and Islam*, Claritas Books, UK, 2023 & *Tranquil Hearts: A Guide to Marriage*, MCAS and MUIS, Singapore, 1998

A well-written book about the effects of pornography which includes various ways we can help those in need. I think the book will add tremendous value to those that are affected by pornography, and will be a useful tool used by professionals to help their clients too.

~ Nasreen Hanifi, Psychologist, Sydney

As a mental health professional, I highly recommend *Porn is Mental* by Wael Ibrahim. This eye-opening book sheds light on the impact of pornography consumption on mental health and well-being. The author presents compelling case studies to illustrate the harmful effects of porn addiction, including anxiety, depression, and relationship problems.

What sets this book apart is the author's approach to the topic. Rather than simply presenting statistics and studies, Ibrahim offers a human perspective by sharing real-life examples of individuals who have struggled with porn addiction. This makes the book relatable and engaging while providing practical advice for those dealing with similar issues. *Porn is Mental* is an essential read for anyone interested in understanding the impact of pornography on mental health.

~ Anna Tajminah Basman, founder of Psycreatives, Mental Health Therapist & Mental Health Coaching

This is a timely book addressing the issues caused by porn addiction within a person's life. Getting help for mental health conditions is becoming easier nowadays and we need to include porn addiction within this. Wael Ibrahim does an excellent job of discussing the harmful effects of porn addiction and the need for mental health professionals to prioritise helping individuals overcome this addiction. This book is useful for everyone to read because porn addiction is something that can affect anyone regardless of age or gender. Knowing the effects of porn addiction can empower you to seek help for yourself or for someone you know.

~ Amirah Zaky, Sex Educator & Vaginismus Coach

This book puts a very strong spotlight on the link between pornography and mental health issues. Regardless how taboo this topic is for many communities, the fact remains that the harm it creates is so significant, especially for our younger generation. I appreciate Sheikh Wael for bringing this issue up so scientifically and comprehensively.

I think this book is relevant to the work of health care clinicians, counsellors, teachers, parents and anyone involved in youth community work. This book is a great tool to use as basis for conversations to reduce the harm of pornography. I hope regulatory bodies can also benefit to take a more serious stance on this issue for the sake of our future generations.

~ Dr Mohammad Gadi, MBBS, FRACGP

DISCLAIMER

I am not a qualified medical doctor, nor have I ever claimed to have the answer to mental health issues, particularly those resulting from porn consumption. What you are about to read in this book is based on recent research and studies that were carefully investigated and backed up by medical practitioners and healthcare professionals from the Philippines and Malaysia.

Consider visiting the references at the end of each chapter if you wish to verify any of the information provided in the book.

Wael Ibrahim

DEDICATION

"To my beloved clients"

CONTENTS

INTRODUCTION

"I can't concentrate on anything; I'm going crazy; I feel like I'm losing my mind; I am depressed; My life is miserable; I feel like ending my life." These are just a few examples of the emails and messages I have been receiving on a daily basis for the past 15 years. All of these emails are typically followed by the phrase "as a result of my addiction to pornography."

In recent years, addiction to pornography has increased at a rate never before seen in the history of humanity. It affects people from all areas of life on multiple levels, including their mental health. With the widespread availability of Internet devices, pornography has also become widely accessible, unmonitored, and unsupervised. People can access pornographic content from the convenience of their homes, offices, school campuses, laptops, tablets, and, of course, mobile devices. Unfortunately, this convenience has led so many people to total dependence on pornographic consumption, in other words, addiction. Undeniably, this addiction is having a profoundly harmful effect on the mental health of millions of people across the globe.

Who would have thought that such imagery would be harmful to our mental health? Who could have imagined that pornography would eventually enslave its consumers and pull them into a lifetime of addiction?

Before going further, I would like to clarify what I mean by addiction.

Addiction is characterized by compulsive behavior including the pursuit of a substance or a specific behavior (*in our context it is pornography*) despite the negative effects it may have on a person's life. To those who are drowned in porn content, does this definition describe what you're going through?

At one point during the course of my research on the harmful impacts of porn, I learned that it can affect brain structure, distort our conception of real sexual intimacy, destroy relationships, have harmful effects on children and adolescents, and so much more. However, I did not anticipate that porn consumption could also ruin people's mental health and lead them to depression, anxiety, and low self-esteem. I never imagined that the detrimental effects of pornography consumption on mental health would be as severe and long-lasting to an extent that in some cases, it is irreversible.

You will learn in the pages ahead, based on considerable research and studies in this field that such explicit images can quickly lead to anxiety, depression, narcissism, low self-esteem, and a multitude of other mental disorders. These significant mental crises that individuals with porn addiction may experience are sometimes indescribable. Numerous porn addicts have expressed a wish to end their life.

Therefore, those who are struggling with porn addiction must seek assistance and support to reclaim their lives and overcome such a devastating addiction in order to better their mental health and the overall quality of their lives.

Ch.1

Porn & low self-esteem

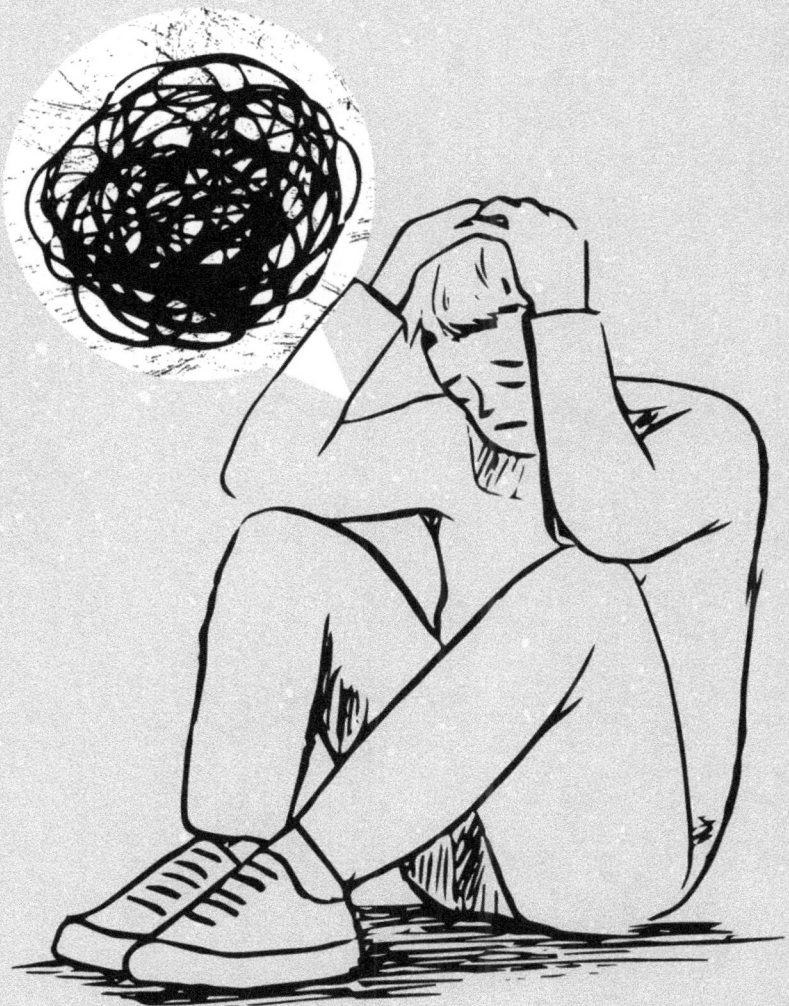

How does porn consumption diminish one's self-esteem?

Key points discussed in this chapter:

[1] Men with low self-esteem are especially drawn to addiction to viewing pornography, as a way to conform to what they think are proper male norms.

[1] Watching scenes that are commonplace in pornography shoots including group sex, orgasms in the face of the female partner, and such, are erroneously viewed as activities that increase self-esteem when in actuality these only contribute to neurochemical pathways of pleasure.

[1] The playboy norms that are depicted in pornographic scenarios are wrongfully viewed as a resource for increasing self-esteem. Men with already low self-esteem are especially vulnerable to this.

[2] Another big aspect of pornography is the issue of the ideal body type. Porn actors and actresses are mainly composed of impossibly fit sthenic mesomorphic body types, with females who are disproportionately voluptuous and men who have lengthy and girthy penises. Realistically, these may not be the proper anatomical feature but it is inevitable for people to have the impression of these body types as the ideal habitus, which may not be practical and clinically applicable to all. This can result in body dysmorphia and affect the self-esteem of regular porn consumers.

[3] Poor self-esteem has been correlated with regular use of pornography, as found in a study. This has also been found to be associated with lower self-worth.

[3] In one study, adolescents who have higher self-confidence were found to have much lesser pornography-seeking behavior.

[4] People with an addiction to pornography were thought to be dealing with self-esteem issues that they are trying to resolve on their own.

Introduction:

As a 15-year-old boy in a local public high school, Felix has been very anxious about his masculinity. Not that he has any doubts about his sexuality, but being surrounded by teenage boys around his age who constantly ramble about their premature sexual escapades puts enormous pressure on him to have a sexual experience himself.

5

His immature mind, not yet geared towards effectively handling information of sexual nature is already pressured to have the sexual experience everybody seems to be having at that age.

One of the primary sources everyone has been talking about are these colorful and extremely graphic websites showing unrealistic bodies of women with voluptuous shapes, highly evident because they have no clothes to cover them. Fueled by a curiosity about what sexual adventures to look forward to, he begins with the search engine and types, "naked women." From at least 25 search attempts in less than an hour, he mentally compiles a number of keywords to search for and website domains to choose from.

Instead of resolving his problems using the information his extensive Internet search has given him, he builds more problems than usual— one of the most confusing of them is, how does he grow to become those men in the videos? When does he achieve his full potential as a man? How does he compare to his classmates according to secondary male characteristics? These questions continue to bother him at present, as a 20-year-old college junior.

This is how pornography affected Felix's self-esteem.

How pornography degrades self-esteem

The people who regularly consume porn convince themselves to have similar primary and secondary sexual characteristics as that of the actors in their favorite pornographic material, thinking that they would achieve better outcomes in their social and sexual relationships. Thinking that pornography would be a good reference for the effective ways to achieve the ideal sex life, people end up consuming pornography as a substitute for the life they want. Instead of viewing pornographic actors as their role models for the sex life they want, they end up being more insecure about their personalities, their bodies, and their overall sexuality. With this in mind, pornography is a double-edged sword that reels one in with pleasure hormones at the cost of gradually decaying self-esteem.

Loss of self-esteem is not the end of how porn degrades the mind. This snowballs to depreciation in the self-worth of the individual. With self-esteem crashing down as they perceive their pornography idols as the standard of perfect sexual characteristics, their self-worth will go down as well. Their identity may also be judged for not having similar physical characteristics as the standard norm of beauty as it is flaunted in pornographic materials. While self-worth is a more general point of view of one's value to the rest of the world, it can be observed directly in a person with the self-confidence that one exudes in their everyday life. Poor self-confidence not only compromises the socio-personal life and real-life relationships of one person but also robs people of opportunities that can offer them a better life. All of these can happen from the mere damage to self-esteem by prolonged pornography use.

Reasons why porn lowers self-esteem

Conforming to the perceived male norms of regularly watching porn. With the growing number of platforms for pornographic content creators, pornography is being established gradually as a well-accepted industry. This industry caters to the common misconception that normal men are supposed to be regular consumers of pornographic content, or they may be demasculinized. They make it seem that the modern male should be aware, if not knowledgeable, of the usual contents of pornographic materials, including names of actors, genres of content, and even famous celebrities with sex scandals. Without this knowledge especially applicable to young males, their peers may perceive them as socially undesirable and not belonging to any group. It can be observed, especially in young children, that shaming kids who do not actively search for sexual content occurs because of the notion that pornographic consumption is part of the male norm.

Therefore, in an effort to conform to the supposed male norms, watching porn is being promoted to be a part of the sex lives of young men. According to a study, men with low self-esteem are especially drawn to addiction to viewing pornography, as a way to belong to the alpha male crowd [1]. This is a common ground that is easy to achieve for people with lower self-esteem with those who have higher confidence, despite having differences in physical attributes, intelligence, and other qualities. Searching for pornographic content seems to equip these men with the knowledge they can use to connect with their intended peers. This is supposed to improve their view of themselves as fully functioning male figures but little do they know, addiction to pornography is both an indication and a cause for much lower self-esteem.

Achieving inconceivable sexual scenarios common in porn content. The pornographic show business industry is famous for creating storylines that are beyond the realm of understanding the reality. Plots that show how easily men can persuade women to engage in sexual acts are almost always in every plot of pornographic videos. Using every line in a book, whether using money, favors or even through blackmail and rape scenes, pornographic scenarios never fail to show the viewers how easy it is for men to convince women to have sex. The thing is, this is not the case in real life.

With these acts being mistaken to be the norm in real-life sexual activity, young inexperienced men are led to believe they can do this in real-life, and upon rejection, experience a significant decline in their self-esteem.

While young men thought that pornographic scenarios are a potential reference on how they can find sexual partners and engage in pleasuring themselves, most of these scenarios are actually fictitious and sometimes presents a threat to the safety and security of their intended partners, which affects the sense of pleasure and satisfaction. In the end, failing to find sexual partners after using pornographic materials as a guide, can further reduce the self-esteem of people, pushing them further into using pornography for sexual satisfaction rather than as a guide to real-life sexual relations with real-life partners. In the end, pornographic content creators win—with every possible reason one could have to use porn, they will use it, regardless of its effect on self-esteem.

The playboy norm. One of the most common scenarios in porn videos is where the actor proceeds to engage with several female sexual partners at a time. With no consequences at all, the male character seems to bask in the benefit of having multiple sex partners, with no strings attached. Not only that, but the scenarios also make it seem that they can do it in a breeze, not requiring any real-life conversational skills or social interactions. The target population in these scenarios vary widely from the people that are close to them such as colleagues, classmates, friends, or even students and in extreme scenarios, family members. These ruin the perception of its consumers regarding the normal dynamics of building relationships in real life. This is the playboy norm, giving inexperienced guys the false idea that the guy can end up with many female sexual partners at a time when finding a single one is difficult already.

The journey to seeking this many female partners can be painful for some guys and can lead to multiple rejections, all of which can further decrease the low self-esteem of men. According to a study, basing social skills and relationship cues on pornography and adapting the playboy norm significantly affects relationship satisfaction, relationship commitment, and even infidelity tendency. Because the plots in pornographic content do not live up to real-life ways of meeting people and building relationships, people who attempt to engage in social relationships based on their expectations from porn end up in unsuccessful encounters. People do not talk the way they talk in pornographic scenes. Women do not normally respond positively to inappropriate attempts of engaging in sexual activity. Most of all, the playboy norm is known to lead to many socio-personal complications, from sexually transmitted diseases to unwanted pregnancies, and risks of infidelity.

"Larger-than-life" aesthetics and anatomy of porn actors. While it is common in pop culture to elevate the classic aesthetics of men and women, such as toned bodies, large bosoms, and girthy penises, these are culturally dependent. For example, in several African countries, girls are force-fed from the age of five years old so that they can grow to have heavier frames and fatter bodies, which are deemed sexually desirable for the men of their culture. In the Western pop culture that is now continuously being adapted to the east, the body image of a pornographic actor lies on classic criteria where the male actor should have a mesomorphic body type, towering height, and a well-endowed penis, which are far from average, while women should have a voluptuous body with ample bosoms and curvy glutes. While these physical features are strongly praised for their beauty standards, some of these characteristics are obtained unnaturally. Men from pornography have huge muscle mass and well-defined body Features which are sometimes a product of taking anabolic steroids to accelerate their muscle growth. Some women working in porn have huge breasts and buttocks as a result of plastic, reconstructive, and aesthetic surgery. In some instances, these physical features may be graphically edited via photo editing software making them more appealing and having them conform to the superior standard of beauty. Because these phenotypes shown in pornography are not all physically or physiologically achievable for all people, some people (especially those who are constantly exposed to pornographic content) turn out to have body image self-consciousness. These people feel more insecure in their bodies and experience negative impacts on their self-confidence, ultimately affecting their self-esteem.

Results of lower self-esteem from porn consumption

While another primary reason for consuming pornographic content is to achieve sexual satisfaction that cannot be achieved through actual sexual intercourse with a partner, several results have been mediated by problematic pornography viewing, one of which is lower self-esteem in their regular consumers. As discussed, pornography has established several standards that are not achievable in the real world, from the physical features of actors and actresses to the social dynamics of casual dating and forming sexual relationships. This eats up the already limited self-esteem of regular porn viewers, which drives them to further consume porn, as opposed to getting out there and mingling with other people.

While this is a grave problem in itself, it also results in further complications from the daily lack of self-confidence, the general decline in overall self-worth, and any further attempts to recover from this state.

1. Lower self-confidence. According to a study, the self-confidence of women constantly exposed to a standard norm of beauty and general physical attributes erode as they see the one-in-a-million facial features and body figures of pornography actresses. They may have the notion that men generally like the physical features of women that one can watch in pornographic videos. This constant pressure for women to adapt to this standard of beauty remains to be a phenomenon that is difficult to justify. Even though it has been constantly reiterated that not all physical features are achievable in most women, there still remains an expectation for women to make efforts to look like women on screen. However, because this is not achievable in most women, their confidence falls even lower as they think of themselves as undesirable.

In addition to this, self-esteem is expected to manifest in the daily actions of a person, which translates to self-confidence. When a person with a perfectly normal body looks constantly at countless pornographic materials with unrealistic physical features, their self-confidence will eventually wear down. This will manifest in how they deal with the people around them and how they form relationships with potential mates. In a study on college students, young adults who were found to have higher self-esteem and self-confidence were also found to have a lower consumption of pornography and its corresponding complications (Pandurang, 2017). A lack of self-confidence can also lead to other deviant behaviors as a coping mechanism, such as increased frequency of taking alcoholic beverages, nicotine addiction, and even use of illicit drugs.

2. Lower self-worth. Addiction to sexual taboos is thought of as one of the most significant reasons for a lack of social acceptance, which lowers overall self-worth (Benoit et al., 2017). This is true not only for regular consumers of porn but also for those who are working in the industry. While their self-esteem is gravely affected due to the much lower respect they may have for themselves, this can translate to a depreciation of their self-worth, especially if they know that they are stuck in the rabbit hole of pornographic addiction. Consuming pornographic content entails different aspects that may be deemed problematic by society. Firstly, masturbation can be frowned upon by various cultures. Since regularly tuning in to porn is highly associated with pleasuring oneself sexually, people who regularly engage in porn consumption are expected to become addicted to masturbation as well, which can be a social taboo in some cultures. Additionally, finding pleasure in unconventional scenarios scripted in porn materials, such as nonconsensual sex, incestuous relationships, and even incorporating pain in the sexual acts, indirectly means consenting, agreeing, and condoning the concepts in the scenes at hand, even if the set-ups are fictitious in nature. And lastly, after reaching the climax when the person is in his logical mindset again not drenched in pleasure hormones, the person may feel guilt and loss of self-respect for finding enjoyment in such porn materials. In this state, the dopamine is too low to regulate the emotional and rational thinking of the individual, further aggravating the loss of one's self-respect and self-worth.

With self-worth being the sense of value given to oneself, it is inevitable that the society around us affects the degree of worth we give ourselves. The decline in self-worth in people who patronize sexual taboos is possibly affected by the inconsistencies of criteria on who is qualified to be worthy of respect in this society. It is the stigma that is given by society to people who take part in culturally unacceptable sexual practices, such as pleasuring oneself while watching extremely graphic sexual content. This is also aggravated by the varying cultures people have in different countries and from different religions, which have contrasting levels of acceptance when it comes to sexually pleasuring oneself. Nevertheless, people who are constantly drenched in sexually graphic materials may lose their respect for themselves.

3. Greater effort for recovery. As opposed to other mental conditions, loss of self-esteem is a factor that can be recovered with the correct treatment, a supportive environment, and an overall proper mindset. In order to recover, the awareness of low self-esteem is vital, as well as finding the source of the problem. While the loss of self-esteem can be perceived almost immediately in most people, the root cause can be difficult to find. And with the neurochemical imbalances brought about by constant pornographic consumption, the brain is not at its peak level to rationalize the root of the problem at hand. In addition to this, while constant pornography consumption is the problem, the people addicted to it ironically see this as their coping mechanism. It will be difficult to get people out of this addiction as long as they see pornography as the solution, and not the problem.

There are some conditions where people can help themselves, such as in the initial phases of overeating or even game addiction. With proper discipline and self-control, they can be saved from getting into the endless cycle of addiction. But for pornographic addiction, it is much more difficult to recover as consuming porn is most probably included in their daily routine and the pleasure that they get from the act cannot be denied. Addictions take intensive discipline and focus to break and replace. With breaking the addiction to pornographic consumption, you'll need to overcome the need to achieve sexual pleasure through the act of watching and masturbating, which by itself is difficult to justify for anyone consumed by porn.

Conclusion

Pornographic materials expose people to content that blurs the practical aspects of sexual relationships and those that are absurdly fictitious. People addicted to porn may think of it as a world where the actors and actresses are the most beautiful and most desirable. In an effort to be like the actors they watch on screen and to have their colorful sex lives, they will try to adopt their image and lifestyle, hoping that they can have satisfying sex lives themselves. They will have unearned confidence to approach the opposite sex, which will likely be socially unacceptable and will result in a failure of connection. Their perception of human connection is tainted by unconventional scenarios from porn. Furthermore, while being unrealistic, these people adopt these impractical standards of beauty and in turn, expect them from everyone, and most of all, from themselves as well. They resort to desperate measures in order to emulate these standards of beauty, which can reach a point where they harm themselves physically and mentally. This creates unrealistic expectations for the people who regularly consume porn and try to emulate it in their lives, which in turn creates disappointing results. Once they realize that they cannot physically reach the standards of beauty that they have set for themselves based on the pornographic actors, their self-esteem will significantly depreciate. Their self-image will be the first to decline. Everything will change including how well they treat themselves. At this point, this will manifest in their everyday lives as a decline in self-confidence which affects their capabilities to engage with other people, form relationships, and even meet people who will truly appreciate their worth. In the long run, this will also affect their overall self-worth as their perception of their value to themselves and to others will depreciate as well. This may translate to how they take care of themselves and how they position themselves in society, whether as a productive member or as someone with less worth. Due to a dissociated view of the world and of themselves as individuals, people who are addicted to porn are at risk of much lower self-esteem.

References:
Borgogna, N. C., McDermott, R. C., Berry, A. T., & Browning, B. R. (2020). *Masculinity and problematic pornography viewing: The moderating role of self-esteem. Psychology of Men & Masculinities, 21(1), 81.*

Kvalem, I. L., Træen, B., & Iantaffi, A. (2016). *Internet Pornography Use, Body Ideals, and Sexual Self-Esteem in Norwegian Gay and Bisexual Men. Journal of Homosexuality, 63(4), 522-540.*

Brown, C. C., Durtschi, J. A., Carroll, J. S., & Willoughby, B. J. (2017). *Understanding and predicting classes of college students who use pornography. Computers in Human Behavior, 66, 114-121.*

Kort, J. (2015). *Pornography, addiction to ("pro"). The International Encyclopedia of Human Sexuality, 861–1042. doi:10.1002/9781118896877.wbiehs360*

Pandurang, MJD. (2017). *Effect of Gender on Self Confidence and Self-Concept Among College Going Students.*

Benoit, C., Smith, M., Jansson, M., Magnus, S., Flagg, J., & Maurice, R. (2017). *Sex work and three dimensions of self-esteem: self-worth, authenticity and self-efficacy. Culture, Health & Sexuality, 20(1), 69–83. doi:10.1080/13691058.2017.1328075*

Ch.2

Porn & social anxiety

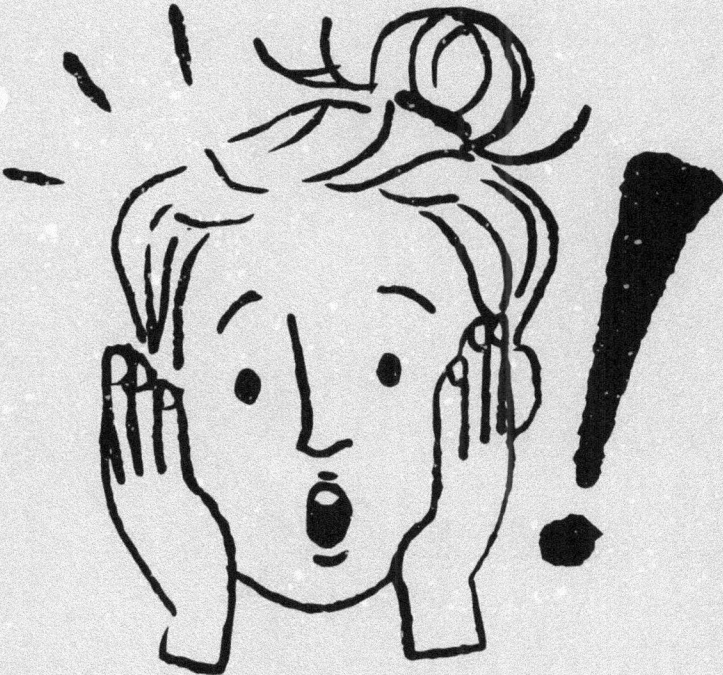

The potential link between porn and social anxiety

Key points discussed in this chapter:

[1] Studies show a correlation between pornography viewing and loneliness, which can be observed by fewer social interactions and the presence of negative emotions.

[2] The resulting social anxiety from mere pornographic exposure results in toxic self-disclosure online, which is further associated with real-life pathologic shyness and a reduction in actual socio-personal connections.

[2] Exposure to sexual images online significantly affects social anxiety and leads to disruptive behaviors, from withdrawal from real-life friends to engaging in risky online behaviors.

[3] Social anxiety does not only affect people who have a pornography addiction but also victims of non-consensual dissemination of sexually explicit media (NCDSEM), who are characters on pornographic material without their consent.

[4] From another perspective, a case study was conducted, showing a possible correlation between the risk of patients with a social anxiety disorder developing hypersexual behavior, and engaging in compulsive sexual activities that are not normally in the habits of the patient.

[4] Developing problematic sexual behavior from a social anxiety disorder patient further weakens the self-control of the patient, which increases the chance of them engaging in risky sexual behavior.

Introduction:

When someone is lonely and bored, what do you think are the possible activities they will do to overcome loneliness? If social contact is not an option due to a pathologic fear of human connection, what does one do? Have you thought of any activities that can simulate human connection without being actually in contact with another individual?

In a normal individual, the ideal answer would be something productive, like playing any sports they love, working out in the gym, or reading some beneficial books. But in a person with social anxiety, the advent of the Internet opened a new world and there is still a lot left unexplored in the World Wide Web.

Young people in their twenties may have the option to lock themselves in their bedrooms and wade into the dark waters of the Internet. For a person with social anxiety who looks at the rest of the population with fear, the Internet is a good place to explore without the risk of running into crippling social interaction. Some may claim to tune in to pornographic sites out of boredom and loneliness. And when boredom becomes a norm in their schedule, then pornography will always be on their list of things they can do to supply much-needed companionship.

The difference between other non-social activities and pornography consumption is that watching pornography has a powerful way of hooking the senses to a neurochemical bliss that is highly addictive—that would make them think that it is as good as the companionship of a real being. In these ways, the consumption of pornography results in a cycle of worsening social anxiety—causing both social disconnectedness and giving them a false sense of security outside the real world where people do indeed talk, care, and interact.

How porn worsens social anxiety

Pornographic consumption affects the capacity of people to conduct social connections in several distinct ways: it can cause social anxiety by allowing a guaranteed boost of pleasure hormones from a pseudo-human connection. This can worsen ongoing anxiety with social connections by inputting deviant behavioral changes that make them less capable of real-life interactions and give other people more reasons to reject and isolate them. In addition to this, people who indulge in pornography seem to dwell on their negative thoughts, even outside of their addiction. Their way of introducing themselves to the world is through toxic disclosure, willingly showing the negative issues in their lives instead of being a positive energy to their colleagues and loved ones. Moreover, pornographic addiction reduces self-control, allowing people, including those with social anxiety, to take part in high-risk behavior. Most worrisome is that this may include hypersexuality, giving them the motivation to participate in high-risk sexual behavior, while having great anxiety when interacting in a normal setting. Furthermore, it can prevent them from seeking treatment, by pulling them further away from the real world.

The cycle of pornographic addiction acts both as a risk factor and an escape for people with social anxiety. They think porn is a coping mechanism in the absence of a social life, however, porn is actually making their condition worse, eventually giving them an excuse to justify their porn-seeking behavior. The following sections explore the effects of constant pornographic consumption on people affected with social anxiety.

Porn precipitates disruptive behavior. Social anxiety disorder entails the irrational fear of scrutiny from people who will be interacting with the person affected. This feeling precipitates when the person with social anxiety thinks they might do something embarrassing in an otherwise normal social situation. No matter how normal any situation is, a person with social anxiety will inevitably overthink and predict and sometimes emulate that they will do something out of the norm. An additional risk factor for social anxiety is pornographic addiction, which can influence the normal behavior of the affected person. While the fear brought about by social anxiety may be out of proportion from the actual threat of embarrassment, adding any disruptive behavior that one may adopt from any porn-curated situations may actually induce real-life shame, a risk for people who regularly watch pornographic materials.

For example, plots in pornographic materials overestimate the level of tolerance of people to sexual allusions, sexually inappropriate cues, and other deviant behaviors. In people who have been an audience of pornographic content for a long time, some sexually inappropriate behavior could become incorporated into their usual actions, which could be deemed disturbing. Even one significant event of shame can elevate the social anxiety of the person, further deviating them away from real-life social interactions, in fear of conducting another embarrassing behavior. When this happens, they will most likely cower back to watching pornography to simulate social, physical, and sexual interactions that they might not have in real life.

The more pressing concern here is that some disruptive behaviors end up as habits that can be more difficult to lose in the long run and can result in further socio-personal complications, such as withdrawal from real-life interactions, worsened fear of social situations, and even a commitment to an unhealthy solitary lifestyle. This offers more reason for people with social anxiety to think of pornography as their escape from these limitations in socializing.

Engagement in porn encourages toxic self-disclosure. Constant exposure to pornographic materials is found to encourage toxic self-disclosure in people with social anxiety disorder, according to one study. With much-limited social interactions in life, these people may have fewer companions in real life to confide in which result in unhealthy outlets for their personal problems. One of these can include online self-disclosure, which is not a reliable outlet for

PORN & Social Anxiety

socio-personal problems because of the variety of personalities of netizens. The problem with this is that the response that they get from people online is not guaranteed to be validating and to be the right answer for their toxic disclosure.

As the comments from people online are not effectively filtered, there is no guarantee that people with social anxiety will receive the help they need from people online. In fact, they can be at risk of various forms of cyberbullying, which will further worsen their social anxiety. These uncalled for responses may include harassment (e.g., when the person sends an offensive message to the person in response to toxic disclosure), outing (e.g., using the personal information that has been disclosed against the person with social anxiety), flaming, (e.g., starting an inappropriate exchange of offensive messages as a response to the toxic disclosure), exclusion (e.g., when the person with social anxiety experiences isolation and singling out due to the toxic self-disclosure done), and masquerading (e.g., bullies creating fake identities and online social media accounts to send offensive messages to the individual and commit other forms of cyberbullying without compromising their true identity).

The usual contents of toxic self-disclosure include irrational fears (e.g., fears that may be perceived as out of proportion from the real-life threat), risky habits (e.g., chronic pornography use, unhealthy sexual practices, etc.), and deviant thoughts (e.g., thoughts of harm towards self or to others), all of which are signs of internal behavioral and pathological struggles.

Porn results in reduced self-control and promotes sexually high-risk behavior. One of the most practical coping mechanisms for the absence of social interaction in individuals with social anxiety is engagement in anonymous online companionship.

Online interactions reduce the level of fear of social interaction in affected people because of physical limitations that remove the demands of actual socialization. In online interactions, eye contact is not required, human touch is absent, and direct verbal interactions are limited. Online interactions provide a perfect medium for people with social anxiety to engage in human interactions, while being a barrier at the same time, as each interaction is masked with anonymity, without any restrictions from standard social regulations, and without any consequence for their deviant behaviors. This can easily turn online interactions into risky encounters, as the anonymity of virtual interaction protects each other's identity, hiding not only their names but also their intentions. This can be prone to varying motivations for anonymous meetings.

This toxic concoction of confounding factors, including anonymity, hidden intentions, loss of accountability, and the sexual nature of the interaction, allows for reduced self-control of people with social anxiety who had found a viable outlet for their intense but obscure sexual energy, without overcoming their dysfunctional fear of human connection. Human interaction in people with pathological social skills can be deemed dangerous as they can have abnormal reflexes from risky situations. They may not know how to react properly in threatening encounters and can put themselves in danger.

The worst-case scenario would be the development of hypersexual behavior, which goes beyond the social conventions of meeting with people, engaging in physical connections, and building relationships. Hypersexuality gives the person unearned confidence of doing sexual activities despite the lack of human connection, which can come off as disrespectful to most people.

Porn use can be used to substitute real-life interaction. The primary limitation of people with social anxiety is their incapacity to form social connections due to pathological shyness. This overwhelming fear of humiliation that is not apparent should have been slowly dissolved with real-life human interaction. In people with pornographic addiction, time spent in front of the screen is precious time that could have been spent with real people forming fruitful relationships. This time spent with others is much needed in people with social anxiety to slowly curb their fear of socializing and help them recover from the devastating psychological distress brought about by their condition. If watching pornography takes time away from friendship, connectedness, and mingling, then people with social anxiety must have found comfort in staying at home, being locked in their rooms, and watching pornography, away from the pressure of socializing. This is especially dangerous when it starts in the critical years of a human's life when they should be gaining their first romantic experience, starting friendships with people with common interests, and building relationships that could last a lifetime.

People who firmly avoid social interactions will find a way to circumvent the need to connect with others. One such way is to resort to pornography for the simulation of the physical and sexual experiences that they will not have in real life. Inherently, they will look for any activity that can give them the experience they crave, without the difficult process of communicating with other people. Because of the nature of pornographic materials, people with social anxiety can be exposed to extensive physical and sexual activities without the need to approach people.

How to reduce social anxiety in porn addicts

Social anxiety and pornography addiction go hand in hand as overlapping problems. Preventing both the habits that entail pornographic addiction, as well as the draining social anxiety, are priorities for the affected people.

Exposure to people. What people with social anxiety mostly dread is that they will commit embarrassing acts while in public. This is probably because these affected people could have spent their early years away from actual people and thus do not know how they interact in real-life situations. One of the places where a person with social anxiety can observe social interactions is in the outdoors. Whether exposure to people occurs in public places such as recreational parks, restaurants, or even public transportation, these people can observe how people interact in real life, without ever needing to have social interactions themselves. They can learn about normal social cues, nonverbal communication, and active listening. They can adapt these social skills and can initiate meaningful connections on their own. At this point, especially early in the experience, the person can limit themselves to listening and observing first, prior to actually using what they have learned and interacting with other people. This can be a less painful experience if the person is with a familiar person, whether a close friend, a co-worker or even a family member, making sure the individual affected does this voluntarily without any form of coercion. Doing so can not only enrich the social skills of people with social anxiety but also give them productive time with their peers, away from watching pornography.

Social skills practice and training. Once they have learned enough social skills from their observations in the exposure phase, they can now apply what they have learned in real life. Finding familiar places to start, they can practice their social skills with their parents, siblings, and even their extended family. These people are great practice buddies for improving communication skills as they are already familiar, so there would be less anxiety around talking to them. In addition to this group, peers at school, work, or in the neighborhood offer familiarity as well. There are times when communication is inevitable, especially in professional and practical instances. Through regular exposure and practice, when the time does come, these people can communicate with others on their own accord, without any assistance.

Social skills have been constantly developing since childhood in normal instances. For those lacking these skills, practice, especially in a supportive environment, can help them improve in confidence and execution. This will also encourage people with social anxiety to turn away from spending time with digital characters from pornographic materials and instead interact with real-life humans and finally build relationships.

Group therapy. An important management for other forms of addiction, including alcohol, nicotine, and illicit drugs, is group therapy. People with very specific roots to their problems may have difficulty finding people who are experiencing the same circumstances as them. Having an addiction to pornography whilst living with social anxiety can be pretty specific, but looking for people with similar problems may be beneficial for them as they would have someone to share their dilemmas in life. A specific protocol is usually instituted for people undergoing group therapy, which entails sharing their experiences with other people affected. This can make people with social anxiety secure, letting them know that there are others experiencing the same issues. In addition to this, as people with social anxiety have difficulty communicating with others, they may find it easier to communicate with people who are just like them, who have the same fears, experience the same difficulties in socializing, and have the same coping mechanisms by pornographic consumption. At the end of the process, people with social anxiety would have found companions, allowing them to practice their social skills amongst themselves. Moreover, spending time with each other means time away from their screens glued to pornographic materials.

Reconnection with friends and family. Reconnecting with people around you may be a challenging feat but can offer a long-term solution to social anxiety and pornographic addiction. Forming real-life connections with family and friends can humanize people and can curb tendencies to seek pornography. Having difficulty doing this when you are experiencing social anxiety is understandable. However, there are several strategies you can use to help overcome your anxiety and improve your relationships with your loved ones. One should gradually expose themselves to social situations with family and friends, starting with small, manageable situations and working their way up to larger events. This can help build their confidence and reduce anxiety. It must also be noted that they must set realistic expectations. It's important to recognize that reconnecting with family members after a period of time apart may not be easy and may take some time, so those affected should be patient with themselves and others.

Dealing with social anxiety can be challenging, especially when it comes to reconnecting with family members. Remember, that it's okay to take things slow and for them to prioritize their own well-being. With time and practice, one can learn to manage social anxiety and build strong, meaningful relationships with family and friends.

Finding other interests. As pornography addiction takes up so much valuable time for people who are addicted to it, it may be strategic to find other interests. Having a habit of resorting to pornography in order to pass time or have a pleasurable activity is detrimental to one's mental health, more so in people with social anxiety. Anyone who has social anxiety aiming to overcome an addiction to pornography, must find other interests or activities to focus on.

One of the most effective activities to raise pleasure hormones in the form of endorphins and serotonin, is exercise. Regular physical activity can help to reduce stress, improve mood, and increase self-esteem, which can be especially helpful in overcoming addiction. Not only can this help people spend time away from their computers and other screens, but it can also improve their physical well-being. Moreover, taking up a new hobby, such as painting, photography, or video editing, which does not exactly require talking to other people, can be beneficial to the person as they can find meaningful activities away from their regular pornographic viewing sessions, without being forced to socialize with the people around them. This can provide a healthy outlet for creativity and help to reduce the urge to view pornography. Also, once they have got out of the habit of viewing porn, they can now be free from the complications of addiction and can gradually find time and have energy to socialize. Taking these steps can improve their overall mental health and wellness.

People who do not respond to such treatment methods may need to consult professional help from psychologists as they know best how to manage both social anxiety and pornography addiction. Talking to a trusted therapist or doctor can be very helpful, as they may have encountered similar instances and have treated these cases from an expert perspective.

References:
[1] Ostrander, M. J. (2021). *Social Anxiety, Pornography Use, and Loneliness: A Mediation Analysis.*

[2] Molavi, P., Mikaeili, N., Ghaseminejad, M. A., Kazemi, Z., & Pourdonya, M. (2018). *Social Anxiety and Benign and Toxic Online Self-Disclosures.* The Journal of Nervous and Mental Disease, 1. doi:10.1097/nmd.0000000000000855

[3] Campbell, J. K., Poage, S. M., Godley, S., & Rothman, E. F. (2020). *Social Anxiety as a Consequence of Non-consensually Disseminated Sexually Explicit Media Victimization.* Journal of Interpersonal Violence, 088626052096715. doi:10.1177/0886260520967150

[4] Okonoda, K. M., & Allagoa, E. L. (2020). *Compulsive Sexual Behaviors in a Young Male with Social Anxiety Disorder (Social Phobia).* Journal of Psychiatry, 23, 471.

Willoughby, B. J., Carroll, J. S., Nelson, L. J., & Padilla-Walker, L. M. (2014). *Associations between relational sexual behaviour, pornography use, and pornography acceptance among US college students.* Culture, Health & Sexuality, 16(9), 1052–1069. doi:10.1080/1369105 8.2014.927075

Ch.3

Porn & Trauma

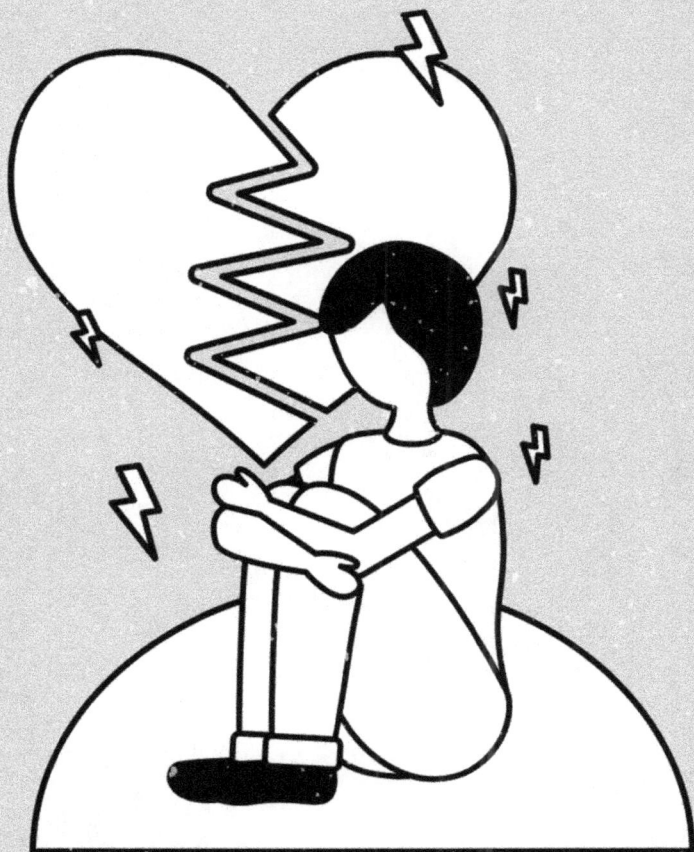

The effects of exposure to pornography on your future

Key points discussed in this chapter:

[1] People who are at risk of developing pornographic addiction are known to likely have a history of childhood trauma, whether from events of physical abuse, or violent events, most especially one with sexual nature.

[1] Determination of pornographic addiction with a nature of childhood trauma can be approached in two ways: through a clinical approach where the person is observed to have symptoms of addiction to sexual engagements, or through a process-based approach where the historical background of trauma and risk factors of the person are meticulously observed and may be correlated to the development of pornographic addiction.

[2] People with an addiction to sexual behavior were also thought to be resolving issues of their own, mostly including childhood trauma.

[2] Multiple studies have also found that adults who grow up to have hypersexual behavior likely have a historical background of sexual abuse during childhood which is likely to be observed to be carried out to adulthood. This can manifest as hypersexual behavior which can also result in the further victimization of more children.

[3] A significant part of the problem in pornographic addicts includes the reenactment of childhood sexual trauma and neglect which they carry over to their adulthood. An alarming concern here is the possibility of conducting the same act of abuse and neglect to children in the lives of adult pornographic addicts. This comes from the premise that trauma victims are observed to re-enact their previous experiences of trauma.

Introduction:

Raquel is an 18-year-old high school senior who is what young people know as popular. While she is revered for her beauty, blonde hair, great smile, and voluptuous body—especially for a teenager—she is not known particularly for her physical image. She is known in the school for being sexually promiscuous and having a particular taste in men who look in their forties and above.

Her personal history suggests that she had brought pornographic materials to her Girl Scout camp in their earlier school years, which was settled internally by their senior Girl Scout mentors and school teachers present in the camp. The case was not brought to the attention of her parents, in the fear that it may cause conflict. No management plans were done and the case was not investigated further. Instead, it spread like wildfire as an unverified rumor throughout her batch mates at school.

Furthermore, she is also rumored to have had a relationship with their guidance counsellor who is a 43-year-old divorced man.

All of these were brought to her mother's attention when the principal called her weeks before their graduation. Anxious but motivated, the principal intently informed Raquel's mother of her escapades and their possible effect on her future as a college student, where youth who are at risk can encounter more similar events. "Ma'am, we are thinking that her past behavior may grow to be a much worse problem in her college years," the principal told Raquel's mom. The mother was utterly confused about what had happened and how all of this occurred without her knowing. Nevertheless, she was straightforward in her solutions and headed to the specialist right away.

Raquel's mum took her to a child psychologist, where it was revealed that Raquel was physically and sexually abused by her uncles, since the age of 11. Since then, Raquel grew to be sexually desirous and stumbled upon pornography on the Internet, growing ever curious. Importantly this took place in the critical part of her development, very early in her puberty. In their first year of high school, she then went to their guidance counsellor. When asked by the child psychologist for the reason for her visit to the guidance office, Raquel confessed to having mixed intentions. She meant to ask for help with her addiction to pornography while being sexually attracted to their (at the time) married guidance counsellor. It seems that the man took advantage of Raquel's vulnerability and groomed Raquel as his young mistress. His wife divorced him after finding out, which gave him more freedom to resume his inappropriate relations with Raquel. Unknown to him, Raquel had several spontaneous sexual encounters throughout her high school life, ranging from classmates to siblings of friends.

Further psychological examining had proven her childhood trauma to have bared her once innocent persona into a bleak woman who is coming of age, but at the wrong pace and with the involvement of the wrong people. Her mind and body are not yet ready for the premature adulthood she had developed early on in her life. Childhood trauma exposes the young mind to concepts that it is not prepared for.

Childhood trauma and pornographic addiction

Pornography has been related to multiple ill events but possibly the most dreadful of them all is the etiology of trauma. In the same way Raquel helplessly became a victim of an unfortunate event in her childhood, most people resort to coping mechanisms to adapt to such traumatic events, especially one that is sexual in nature. Raquel was in a particularly vulnerable stage of her life, being gravely under-aged while being at the receiving end of abuse from someone who she should be able to trust.

The severity of the damage to her is caused by a myriad of risk factors. At a very early age, she experienced a violating event, which her young mind cannot process yet, in addition to a fairly new physical sensation to her, which blurs the line between violence and pleasure. Her rational mind also possibly had not processed yet that what occurred to her was morally, socially, and legally inappropriate. Her mind failing to find a resolution to this event has encouraged her to seek answers, which in the case of a young person living in the modern world meant searching the Internet for similar cases. With no one to guide her on how to recover from what happened, she let her environment and curiosity take over, showing her more similar scenarios in the form of pornographic videos. The risk factors of a young immature mind, uninformed rationality, and a bruised body with a demoralized soul, all at an early age, did not help her recover from this childhood trauma.

Unresolved childhood trauma and seeking answers in pornography

Children usually seek explanations on their own on how to justify the events that transpired every time they encounter a traumatic event. This is difficult because in sexual abuse cases which are undocumented and unreported, there is usually no accountability to the abusers, which leaves the problem in the open. This leaves no one to rationalize what happens to the victim, making them think about and resolve things on their own, without assistance from others.

As they may not know the reason why they were abused, they tend to seek reasons, even the most irrational ones. Whether they are unloved, they deserved to be hurt, or they indeed found pleasure in the activity. From the perspective of the abuser, victim blaming can be part of the mechanism, as the abuser tries to justify their malicious actions. Some state that it is the clothes of the victim that make them attractive and at risk of being a victim of sexual harassment and abuse. Some even state that they are receiving sexual cues from the victim. Regardless of the intention and how it happened, sexual abuse will leave a confusing scar in the victim's memory.

The fuel for curiosity in victims of child abuse is the unresolved childhood trauma. As the child knows that the events can be recalled in sex videos and similar materials, they may start seeking answers in pornography. This way, the victim need not confide to other people what had happened but just visualize the abuse through the recalling of the abuse but in pornographic videos.

Trauma and hypersexuality

Pornography offers visualization of what transpired in a potentially blurry traumatic event, especially for those who experienced them firsthand at an early age. Knowing that the plots of pornographic films are fictitious, exaggerated, and, at most times, inappropriate, these pornographic materials are not the best media to teach sex to young people. But for the victim of trauma, pornography offers several solutions.

Pornography allows the person to visualize what possibly could have transpired in a sexually distressing event. While the real traumatic experience is highly likely to be painful and violent in nature, the mind sometimes has the tendency to protect oneself from this pain by blocking the memory of the details of the event and sometimes creating false memories, which further tickles the curiosity of the victim for an explanation. Pornographic media curates a wide range of sexual content, even tapping into the more violent scenarios, which may contain images that the victim is inadvertently seeking.

In studies, most hypersexual people have been probed to have had a history of childhood trauma that is sexual in nature. A possible explanation would be the creation of a coping mechanism to substitute pleasure with the anxiety from the trauma. The mind may have resorted to pornography for a dopamine boost that makes the victim forget the traumatic event just for several moments. Because this is not a permanent solution to the psychological scars, the victim will seek more porn and the pathophysiology of addiction will take over. The habits of these hypersexual people are almost gravely effective as the addictive dopamine is regularly sought after every day of their lives. At this phase, it is easy to fall into pornographic addiction, giving these victims of trauma the much-needed dopamine boosts, with just the click of a link.

Childhood trauma and shame

According to a study, childhood trauma is a significant factor in perpetuating sexual compulsivity in people who are victims of abuse. This could be on top of having post-traumatic stress disorder, secondary to traumatizing experiences such as neglect, sexual abuse, and physical maltreatment.

In children who grew up without the proper guidance of their parents, older siblings, or any other guardians, childhood trauma cannot be handled well by a young mind. The immature mind interprets trauma in various ways. Some children blame themselves for the traumatic event, thinking that they must have deserved the abusive actions. In most children, the traumatic event is well-imprinted on their minds, replaying over and over again, in an endless loop of rumination, which in turn brings back the feeling of fright upon induction of a stimulus, such as a touch, hearing familiar noises, or a sighting of a similar event.

This can be highly relevant especially if the sexual abuse has been done to the child repeatedly, imprinting a stronger memory on the child. Whatever the mechanism is, the repeated rumination of the event will have to be resolved somehow and one of the endgames of this is the feeling of guilt. In these instances, the person may feel guilt, not only because they may have done something wrong to deserve the abuse, but also because the event may have a pleasurable aspect as the nature of abuse is sexual. This could eventually lead to shame, in which the victim may feel the need to be covered up by something that can substitute the feelings of sexual satisfaction, without the hurt. With today's accessibility online, pornography addiction could easily be something to cover the shame.

Shame serves as a barrier to recovery. As the mind will try to protect the individual from another event, the guilt may not recover readily in these people. In the end, the significant history of childhood trauma, the shame one person may have felt from it, and the resulting sexual compulsivity, all form a powerful triad that enforces pornography addiction.

Pornography as a coping mechanism

Others are able to coop up their sexual energy without releasing it in any aggressive forms, they may find other outlets for this tension. Traumas of the sexual kind usually lead to a coping mechanism that is sexual in nature as well. The greater the weight of the sexual trauma on the child, the more intense the urge of the person to resort to finding carnal relief.

Other victims of sexual trauma have a psychological coping mechanism known as blocking, where the brain subconsciously forgets other memories that can hurt the individual. Nevertheless, the brain forces the individual to cope with the abuse somehow, which can encourage the person to adopt a habit that can cover the shame they are feeling. Despite forcefully forgetting the abusive event, the sexual tension remains unreleased and undefined of its intentions.

This is where pornographic addiction takes place, when in the click of a button, the victim of abuse can induce a pleasurable experience without any of the pain that they have received from the event of the sexual abuse. Pornographic addiction is one of the adult sequelae of childhood trauma and sexual abuse. And while other problems can be solved easily by tackling the root cause, childhood abuse may not be resolved readily as the traumatic event has happened already and can never be reverted back.

Pornography and trauma reenactment

The immense childhood trauma can trigger a person's desire to find a point of relief, which can lead to any form of addiction. In some victims of abuse, rumination is not sufficient to recall and resolve the events of the abuse. Trauma reenactment can take place in some of the worse sexual abuse cases, which further increases the number of victims of abuse.

In multiple studies, juvenile criminals are highly likely victims of sexual abuse as children, with much worse outcomes in unreported cases. This can lead to behavior mirroring the abuse they have experienced before as children, which they can reenact to new victims, making it a form of secondary sexual hostility. In some cases of sexual abuse conducted by adults, thorough history can be evaluated to check if that same criminal was once an abused child as well. This constitutes the cycle of abuse, which if unresolved would result in horrific consequences in the form of sexual aggression.

Trauma reenactment cannot always be conducted, depending on the victim. While some may resort to sexual offense to others, others have the self-control to prevent themselves from hurting anyone else. Despite the better outcomes in sexual abuse victims who do not end up as criminals, they must find another coping mechanism to adapt to the feeling of sexual tension that they could not release in a partner of a consenting relationship. Pornographic content can easily be accessed to reenact the sexual act visually and through the rich imagination of the person. This could easily become a habit because these people justify their porn addiction as a coping mechanism to sexual abuse, rather than committing a criminal offence. This can also be observed in places with higher socioeconomic status, where instead of committing sexual harassment and abuse, people resort to pornography to release their sexual energy.

Attachment failure in pornography addicts

One of the long-term sequelae of pornographic addiction in victims of childhood abuse is attachment failure. Victims of abuse need social support the most. It should be understood that being in a functional relationship can help them recover from both childhood trauma and pornographic addiction. But with the corresponding complications of both, affected people may have problems committing to real-life relationships. To start with, their basic human and emotional needs are much different from people who are not in some kind of addiction and do not have a history of trauma.

While other people with normal socio-personal development can catch up to the average needs of the person as required by societal, environmental, and personal factors, porn addicts with a history of sexual abuse need a resolution from their mental anguish, which has been unresolved since childhood. This requires a different management plan, apart from opening up, talking about it, and forming companionship with people who can understand their situation. This can entail medical and psychological management, which can be too much for an average person who just wants a normal life. Most people cannot understand these needs and thus may not last long in relationships with people who have an addiction to pornography.

Intimacy problems in trauma victims

Intimacy problems are one of the most pronounced problems of victims of sexual abuse. Victims of sexual abuse have varying degrees of guilt and shame from the trauma that they have experienced. This can induce flashbacks of the sexual abuse, which can interfere with their intimate relationship with others as adults.

Some resort to pornography to normalize their sexual acts and form healthy sexual relationships with their romantic partners. The problem is that pornography is not the best resource for an ideal sexual relationship as it entails fictitious, unrealistic, and definitely unhealthy practices. Victims of abuse may end up being more dependent on pornography than forming actual healthy intimate relationships. At some point, dependence may become an addiction, which crosses the fine line between love and lust.

Pornography addiction has a peculiar way of removing the romantic aspect of sexual intimacy. In pornography addicts, the sexual taste can be significantly altered as influenced by the content they consume from pornographic materials, which can then be manifested as a different and possibly abnormal interest not applicable in a normal romantic and sexual relationship. This can be found in a lack of the romantic aspect of the sexual relationship of a couple, which can be simultaneously influenced by their addiction to pornography and their history of sexual abuse.

Nevertheless, in desperate attempts to find real intimacy, some victims of sexual abuse may wrongfully resort to pornography for resources on sexual references. In other victims of sexual abuse who have resorted to porn addiction as their coping tendency, they may encounter intimacy problems as their sexual arousal may be dependent on pornographic content only as opposed to actual physical stimuli.

Whatever the circumstance is, victims of sexual abuse have their brains rewired completely differently and possibly irreversibly, which can affect their adaptations to sexual stimuli. These victims can resort to pornography to cover up guilt and shame, to justify the sexual tension they are feeling, or even to look for references to regain sexual intimacy with their current romantic partner.

References:

[1] Wéry, A., Schimmenti, A., Karila, L., & Billieux, J. (2018). Where the mind cannot dare: a case of addictive use of online pornography and its relationship with childhood trauma. Journal of Sex & Marital Therapy, 1–35. doi:10.1080/0092623x.2018.1488324

[2] Kort, J. (2015). Pornography, addiction to ("pro"). The International Encyclopedia of Human Sexuality, 861–1042. doi:10.1002/9781118896877.wbiehs360

[3] Griffin-Shelley, Eric (2014). Sex and Love Addicts, Who Sexually Offend: Two Cases of Online Use of Child Pornography (Child Sexual Abuse Images). Sexual Addiction & Compulsivity, 21(4), 322–341. doi:10.1080/10720162.2014.966936

Ch.4

Porn & mental conditioning.

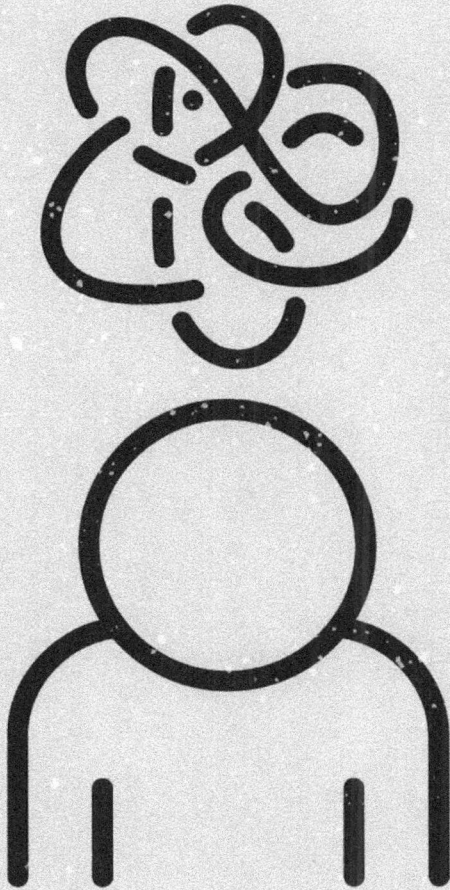

The psychological blockage and inability to sexual performances (PIED)

Key points discussed in this chapter:

[1] Erectile dysfunction has long been known to be potentially induced by excessive use of pornography, as there is a mental shift in sexual stimuli in the erection of men with such sexual problems. This is known as pornography-induced erectile dysfunction (PIED).

[1] Withdrawing from using internet-based stimuli to induce erection and orgasm has been found to affect men with erectile dysfunction positively, as the sexual stimuli can be unlearned. However, this feat is incredibly difficult especially for pornography addicts, as the use of sexual multimedia materials from the internet is already programmed as their stimuli for sexual function.

[1] An additional problem in people with pornography addiction is the pathologic difficulty in achieving orgasm with a real-life sexual partner, which decreases the pleasure in the man afflicted and affects the satisfaction of his partner as well.

[1,2] In addition to problems with erectile dysfunction, the libido, in general, has been significantly affected in the subjects of studies who are known to have an addiction to pornographic use. This is known as pornography-induced abnormally low libido. Low sexual desire has been a devastating effect of pornography due to different reasons. Pornographic materials can create unrealistic expectations when it comes to sexual experience and may decrease the standard level of satisfaction of one person.

[3] According to a study, men who have a general preference for achieving orgasm through masturbation with internet pornography materials than in physical sexual intercourse with a partner are found to have increased sexual dysfunction, which further proves that the frequent exposure and utilization of online sexual multimedia materials affect the overall sexual function.

[4] While advanced age used to be the determining risk factor of erectile dysfunction in men, it was found according to studies that the incidence and prevalence of erectile dysfunction in younger men has been correlated to their increased pornographic consumption.

Introduction:

Leandro, thinking he's like any other 13-year-old out there, has adopted the habit of masturbating every morning, before going to shower. This was the time he got his very own personal desktop in his own room. No matter how early he has to be up for school, he would get up much earlier to make time for his morning fix. "I do it because, I have the morning wood, and it would be awkward to walk around our house with it," Leandro confessed to me, as he tries to justify his regular morning habit. In fact, he does not have to, because his morning wood is gone after urinating in the morning. Nevertheless, he does it every day with no miss.

He gets up very early in the morning to masturbate, then sleeps late at night to do it again. He emphasizes that he does not miss any important responsibility because of this habit, as he always makes sure that he has done all of his homework, house chores, and even feeding his birds. It has become a normal activity for him, an important part of his lifestyle, and a way to start and end the day.

Up until adulthood, Leandro adopted the habit of masturbating right before taking a shower even without the morning wood. He came to accept that it is part of his day, even though he is not sexually aroused by anything. Sexual desire is not there anymore, it's more like a scheduled activity. It has become an addiction or a very strong habit. "It was pleasurable once, especially during my teenage years. We as teenage boys used to exchange porn videos with our friends," he explained.

"Have you ever experienced that whenever you feel bored, you will look up at the fridge to see if you can eat something, though you are not necessarily hungry, but just bored? You can feel your body

PORN & Mental Conditioning

just automatically walks to the fridge and involuntarily opens the fridge door, searching for anything to chew on but without any complete conscious thought. It's how I feel about masturbation," he confessed. "The problem is, I have my wife now and whenever we have sex, I can't seem to get *it* up. Having a wife who actually needs to have someone to share the sexual energy with, it is now much more difficult to adjust my sexual needs, more than ever."

The issue was brought to light when he asked for medical consultation with a urologist, regarding erectile dysfunction. He did not expect it but he was also referred to a psychologist, in addition to some pharmacologic management for his erectile dysfunction.

The psychologist had come to the conclusion that pornography addiction had done some extensive mental conditioning for him, replacing his normal sexual stimuli, such as touch or scent, with artificial stimuli from pornographic content, such as very graphic visual cues and exaggerated auditory cues. Leading to the experience of pleasurable masturbation instead of the supposedly sexual pleasure with his wife. Not only that, but his sexual taste has also significantly changed.

Leandro has never been this confused. He claims and asserts to always achieve erection regularly because he masturbates to porn every day. He also never thought of consuming porn as an addiction, and instead thought of it as something like watching his regular TV series every day. He claims to have never been affected by it. But what he did not realise is that his daily habit has reprogrammed his brain to favor graphic, or rather pornographic content over humanly physical touch.

Mental conditioning in pornography addiction

Leandro is a classic victim of mental conditioning brought about by regular exposure to pornographic content. This had programmed his brain to respond differently from the caressing touch of his wife, making that a neutral stimulus as compared to the highly graphic sexual materials on the Internet.

Mental conditioning is a process of imposing a neutral stimulus as a positive trigger of a particular action or outcome. In people who have a porn addiction, the mind is conditioned to respond with immediate arousal on auditory and visual cues from pornography materials, whether it's a viral sex video from the Internet or an arousing story on the escapades of a nymphomaniac. The person induces arousal through the physical touch of the erogenous zones in the body while watching, reading, or listening to pornographic content, which trains the brain to be sexually excited upon receiving artificial sexual stimuli. This does three things. It affects the natural mechanism of sexual arousal, it makes it difficult for the people affected to maintain a stable penile erection, and it usually results in an unsatisfying sexual climax.

The habit of consuming pornography is what started all of this. It is difficult to lose a habit, especially one that soaks your brain in pleasure hormones. For people like Leandro, the rational mind says that masturbating to porn is not important to your morning lifestyle, but they do it anyway. It's automatic. As a result, mental conditioning takes place naturally, shifting the things that arouse them, changing their sexual taste, and eventually numbing their brain to pleasure.

Porn-induced erectile dysfunction

Problems with maintaining erection also significantly manifest after a certain amount of pornography consumption. Mental conditioning limits the duration of erection in physical sexual activity due to the ineffective sexual stimuli without the pornographic material, and because during masturbation, the hand is likely assisting the male member almost the entire time, which does not reflect the same stimuli for the sex organ during actual intercourse. The brain recognizes when the individual himself touches and holds his own body parts, as opposed to when another person induces the physical touch. This difference contributes to the maintenance of erection throughout the sexual activity.

Erectile dysfunction has long been known to be potentially induced by excessive use of pornography, as there is a mental shift in sexual stimuli in the erection of men with such sexual problems. The brain does not respond to the usual sexual stimuli even at varying degrees of exposure.

One can observe this upon attempting to get into a stable relationship after years of dependence on pornography for sexual satisfaction. Even with the appropriate physical sexual stimuli from a consenting partner, the affected guy may not sexually achieve arousal. Different physical approaches may be done but will not institute erection on the part of the guy. Sexual arousal, which is needed to initiate and conduct a sexual activity with a partner, may be initiated by visual stimuli, physical stimuli, or even auditory stimuli, but may be affected by long-term pornography addiction. This is known as pornography-induced erectile dysfunction (PIED) [1].

Difficulty in inducing arousal

In addition to difficulty in maintaining an erection, this disturbs the natural mechanism of sexual arousal in humans, substituting humanly erotic touch from a sexual partner or possibly the scent of the pheromones from the people you are sexually compatible with, with computer-derived sexually graphic materials. What this means is, even in the event of an actual sexual activity, a guy may not be able to achieve an erection, even with the caressing touch from their sex partner, but instead would need to watch pornographic videos to achieve arousal. This is what happened to Leandro when actual physical touch becomes downgraded to a neutral stimulus for his sexual arousal.

This is usually a result of the changing stimuli received during porn consumption versus during actual sex with a partner. Watching pornography online gives a different set of triggers for arousal, such as sounds of exaggerated moans from the porn actors or the sighting of visual cues by the unrealistic body features of porn actors. Like different people who have different triggers, every porn addict has different combinations of erotic stimuli that floods one's urges to watch and achieve arousal to porn. This can promote the highly graphic audiovisual cues as the sexual prompt for the porn addict, as opposed to the stimuli that most likely occurs in the physical setting, such as the scent of your partner and the playful fondling of the erogenous parts. For a porn addict intending to relearn how to find pleasure in a humanly sexual encounter, one must compare these very specific urges they have while they are watching pornography versus the normal sexual cues with an actual sexual partner.

Inability to reach climax

According to studies, 45 percent of young adult men who are chronic porn consumers have been experiencing erectile dysfunction that affects their overall sexual satisfaction. Seeking consultation from specialists usually comes from the most common chief complaints of the patients affected, which is another one of the most problematic outcomes of PIED, which is the difficulty of reaching orgasm [1].

Even on a real-life sexual partner, the sexual stimuli seem to be not enough to induce sufficient pleasure to reach the climax of one sexual arousal. This is already a combination of pathology in the neurochemical and possibly the urogenital organs, as the body is now used to being dependent on pornographic material to achieve sexual satisfaction. Without any obscene visual and auditory stimuli from any pornographic material, the brain seems to not release the neurochemical signals to achieve the much-needed sympathetic response of the autonomic nervous system that will trigger the orgasm. This results in frustration on the man's part, dissatisfaction on the woman's part, and potentially a conflict within their overall relationship.

While this is only a part of the problem, this constitutes the main dilemma of men, especially ones in a long-term romantic relationship as anejaculation can cause insecurities in both partners. The inability to reach climax can be a multi-factorial problem, which can include loss of sexual attraction to the partner, lack of physical capacity to reach the climax or even an overall loss of sexual desire. But in many cases, porn addiction can be the root cause of the problem.

Problems with ejaculation and reaching orgasm

Sexual satisfaction is not optimally achieved during physical sexual activity with a partner. Problems with feeling arousal and maintaining an erection can contribute to the overall pleasure the guy receives during a sexual activity, as well as their partner's. In some cases, the male does not reach the climax, limiting his capacity to orgasm and worse, can eventually encounter difficulties with ejaculation. These are now a combination of neurological, psychological, and hormonal problems, effectively weaved by years of pleasuring oneself to pornographic materials.

Anejaculation or the complete inability to ejaculate is one of the dreaded complications of pornography addiction. When the sexual response of the individual is highly dependent on porn content, it will be very difficult to ejaculate due to an unintended hesitancy by your autonomic nervous system, which controls the involuntary mechanism of reaching orgasm. In these cases, orgasm can be achieved by releasing little to no seminal fluid. In worse cases, anorgasmia can happen, where there is completely no orgasm achieved after a through rigorous sexual intercourse. These cases can reflect the overall satisfaction of the people affected.

In some cases, the male forces themselves to ejaculate once the sensation is apparent, but this can come off as an ineffective one. Retrograde ejaculation can happen when the semen is transmitted to the bladder instead of out of the penis, which can be observed as little to no semen release. Though this is rare, exerting enough pressure to release semen can instead open the bladder sphincter which can receive the semen, instead of being directing through the penile urethra. The lack of seminal volume can affect the overall sense of satisfaction in men, as well as their partners. In men who have difficulty achieving orgasm, they tend to try harder and extend the sexual intercourse, in an effort to achieve climax for both partners. In these cases, sexual intercourse can extend for longer periods of time and can be tiring, thus affecting overall satisfaction. This happens usually in cases of delayed ejaculation, where the male partner still attempts to reach orgasm, despite prolonged intercourse.

Declining libido

While regular pornographic use seems to reflect the libido of the man, this is not always the case. For chronic pornographic consumption, the neural pathways in the brain and the peripheral nerves to the reproductive organs are not what they used to be, demanding a different rate and kind of sexual stimuli and having a dysfunction in sex hormones as a response to normal sexual stimuli induced by a live partner. This reflects another problem in the afflicted patients, where, the libido, in general, has been significantly affected in the subjects of studies who are known to have an addiction to pornographic use. This is known as pornography-induced abnormally low libido.

Low sexual desire is a devastating effect of pornography. Pornographic materials can create unrealistic expectations when it comes to sexual experience and may decrease the standard level of satisfaction of one person. So after years of regular use of pornography, the real-world physical stimuli may not be good enough anymore.

In the human body, libido normally declines with a lack of specific hormones, problems with the reproductive system, or even due to systemic illnesses. In addition to these, mental health issues can significantly affect libido including worsening depression, anxiety, and stress. Relationship issues can also affect the sexual desire one individual has for their partner. While some of these are physiologically expected in the body, some risk factors are actually preventable. In people who are chronic porn consumers, libido is expected to crash over the years, possibly due to dependence on porn and tolerance to pleasure hormones. Addiction is a significant part of the decrease in libido, not only in porn but also in other factors inducing dopamine flooding. Substance abuse can also contribute to the waning libido of people, including increased alcoholic beverage intake, chronic nicotine exposure, and intake of illicit drugs. All of these, on top of the porn addiction problem, can significantly aggravate the decrease in libido.

Getting out of mental conditioning

Pornography-induced mental conditioning of stimuli for sexual response can be reversed over time. With proper management, therapy, and consistency, mental conditioning can be reverted back. This may take intensive dedication and self-discipline.

Awareness of triggers for watching porn is always the starting point in treating this addiction. The first step is to become aware of their mental conditioning and identify the limiting beliefs and thought patterns that are holding them back. Being aware of the mechanism from sexual stimulus to reaching orgasm, one can watch their thoughts and see if they can consciously fight the urge to masturbate with the artificial stimuli for arousal.

In the case of Leandro, the important thing is that he is aware of his urges. But for many, awareness is very difficult to realize. Many people who have porn addiction would deny their addiction and try to justify their actions. If this cannot be achieved by an individual, it is ideal that people around him can notice. In cases of erectile dysfunction, their partners can respectfully inform the affected individual so that they can seek help if needed.

Awareness of other problems is important. Performance anxiety is common in people who are chronic porn consumers as they may have latent insecurities about what they have usually watched. In people who have issues with their current sexual partner, this must be cleared as it can contribute to porn-induced erectile dysfunction. Additional problems one needs to be aware of include emotional problems, such as depression, anxiety, and stress.

It is also important to question one's beliefs by challenging the validity of their reasons for consuming porn and by asking questions like "Is this really necessary?" and "Do I deserve the consequences of addiction in my life?"

Substituting actions can effectively replace porn consumption if done right. Seeking new experiences entails trying new things out and exposing oneself to different perspectives, cultures, and ideas. This will help broaden your horizons, challenge your preconceived notions, and eventually veer you away from consuming pornography.

For some, prayers and being faithful to one's religion is also a proven way to connect oneself to what they want to be as a person. Engaging in religious duties and spiritual practices can help develop greater self-awareness and increase your ability to respond to challenging situations that test self-discipline against addiction in a flexible and adaptive manner.

Surrounding oneself with supportive people can help the affected individual veer themselves away from pornography by humanizing people, as opposed to seeing them as characters in pornographic material or as sex objects. Seeking out people who inspire and encourage a person to grow and expand one's thinking would encourage affected people to find companionship instead of locking themselves away from the rest of the world. One must avoid spending time with those who reinforce their limiting beliefs and thought patterns.

References:
[1] Park, B., Wilson, G., Berger, J., Christman, M., Reina, B., Bishop, F., ... Doan, A. (2016). Is Internet Pornography Causing Sexual Dysfunctions? A Review with Clinical Reports. Behavioral Sciences, 6(3), 17. doi:10.3390/bs6030017
[2] Dwulit, A. D., & Rzymski, P. (2019). The potential associations of pornography use with sexual dysfunctions: An integrative literature review of observational studies. Journal of Clinical Medicine, 8(7), 914.
[3] Berger, J. H., Kehoe, J. E., Doan, A. P., Crain, D. S., Klam, W. P., Marshall, M. T., & Christman, M. S. (2019). Survey of sexual function and pornography. Military Medicine, 184(11-12), 731-737.
[4] Jacobs, T., Geysemans, B., Van Hal, G., Glazemakers, I., Fog-Poulsen, K., Vermandel, A. ... & De Win, G. (2021). Associations between online pornography consumption and sexual dysfunction in young men: multivariate analysis based on an international web-based survey. JMIR Public Health and Surveillance, 7(10), e32542.
Park, B. Y., Wilson, G., Berger, J., Christman, M., Reina, B., Bishop, F., ... Doan, A. P. (2016). Is internet pornography causing sexual dysfunctions? A review with clinical reports. Behavioral Sciences, 6(3), 17.

Ch.5

Porn & Depression

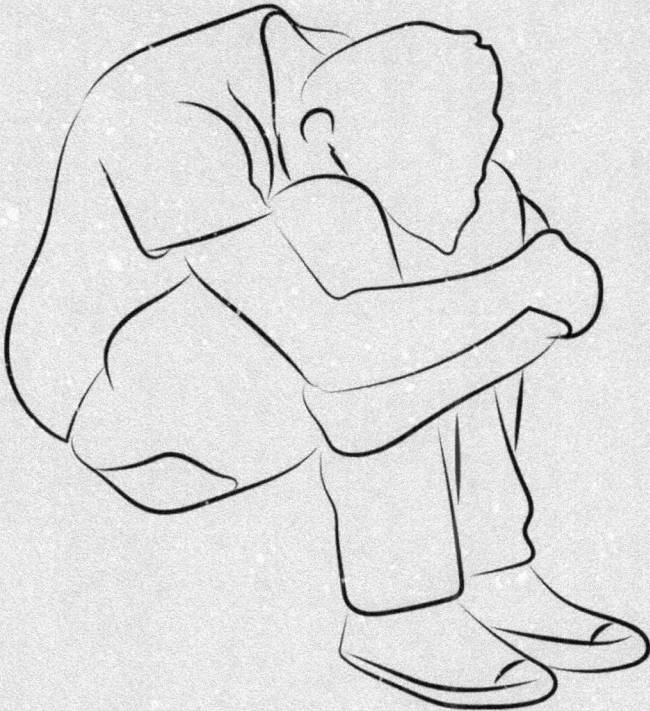

Depressive symptoms & suicide attempts

Key points discussed in this chapter:

[1] Regular pornographic consumption has been associated with negative mental health implications as confirmed by various studies. As a matter of fact, people who frequently view sexually explicit materials online have been found to have higher risks for depression.

[1] In people who had been diagnosed with clinical depression, symptoms have been far worse upon frequent consumption of pornographic materials.

[1] In people with depression, the use of pornography has been thought to be used for self-regulation of negative emotions that are bothering them as symptoms of depression. Coping with depression can be difficult for people, especially with the limited acceptance of mental health problems in certain cultures, which makes it difficult to look for healthy coping mechanisms. With the presence of sexually explicit material being more accessible than ever, it has been the option for more and more people, which leads to further disruption of neurotransmitter balance in their depressed minds.

[2] One of the most remarkable findings of studies looking for risk factors for depression in pornographic users is their perception of porn as conflicting with their moral beliefs. According to a study, men who were found to be conflicted pornography consumers, meaning they think watching pornography is wrong, but still proceed to consume it, are at significant risk of developing symptoms of clinical depression, as opposed to their counterparts who do not believe that watching porn is wrong.

[3] A similar study also proves how scrupulosity affects the risk of porn viewers developing depressive symptoms as these people have feelings of moral conflict at the back of their minds while engaging in pornographic consumption.

Introduction:

Dysphoria, or as we commonly known it, the depressed mood, is the negative mood serving as an adaptive emotional response to disappointment, loss, or failure. When these signs and symptoms form a constellation of clinical presentations, both psychological and physiological in nature, then they can be qualified as depressive syndromes, further classified as major depressive disorder, minor depression, or persistent depressive disorder. In the United States, there is an expected lifetime prevalence of major depression of over one-fifth of the population (21 percent), not accounting the unreported and undocumented cases. Worldwide, the lifetime prevalence of major depression is at 5 percent, while persistent depressive disorder is at a higher rate of 12 percent. The average age of onset was found to be at 30 years old, implying that possible long-term problems have been encountered in the earlier years of life, such as emotional turmoil, life challenges, or even disruptive habits – which is where pornographic addiction comes in to play.

Pornographic addiction has been found to be one of the increasingly significant risk factors contributing to depression, especially in the advent of much better accessibility to the World Wide Web, putting the depressed person at further risk for higher stress, anxiety, and even suicide ideation. This could be further aggravated by other risk factors such as having a dysfunctional family, unstable source of income, and even problematic relationship status. Because of what porn does to the brain, chronic use of pornography also puts the depressed person at risk of other mental disorders such as anxiety disorders and panic disorders. Pornography plays different roles in the mechanism of depression in affected people.

Porn as a risk factor and an etiology of clinical depression

According to studies, porn dependence is a strong risk factor for negative mental health status, one of which is depression. In people who have been using pornography for a long time, the risk of having any form of depressive disorder is much higher than in a non-dependent individual [1]. The prevailing problem today is that the length of time measured in using pornography is growing, as the average age of early porn exposure is now 10 years old, based on statistics. This would probably be expected to be a regular activity after several months of use, which would then be a difficult habit to lose. Because of how pornography rewires the brain and disrupts its pleasure centers, the much-needed dopamine for curbing depression is not efficient anymore, making chronic porn use a significant risk factor for depressive disorders, including other negative mental health problems.

In people who are already diagnosed with clinical depression while being dependent on pornography, the symptomatology is much worse than in a depressed patient without regular use of porn, according to a study. This puts us into a perspective of how the usage of pornography is directly correlated with the incidence and worsening manifestations of clinical depression. Because of varying motivations of people to use porn due to depression, it is difficult to justify to them why it is doing more harm than good and thus is expected to stay in their lifestyle despite its documented effects on their mental status.

The pathophysiology of depression and pornographic addiction

For people who start out with a normal mental disposition, constant pornography consumption soaks the brain in pleasure hormones, which entails a self-induced spike in dopamine. While this is normal in response to sexual activity, obtaining dopamine surges and pleasure response from porn is different as it increases the tolerance of the brain to the neurotransmitter, thus requiring higher amounts of dopamine whenever it's needed. The problem is that dopamine is not only required for sexual satisfaction but for emotional regulation as well, such as when handling episodes of sadness, anxiety, and disappointment. In the long run, when the person reaches addiction to pornographic consumption, they will have dysfunctional dopamine release and reception for emotional regulation, putting them at risk for depression.

For people who are depressed already to start with, pornography may serve as a coping mechanism to make up for the sadness that they are feeling, thinking that pleasure can offset the depressed phase that is burdening them. They treat their porn watching sessions as an adaptive reaction to feeling down, as they numb their feelings with short-term pleasure and self-induced sexual satisfaction. The problem with this is that since dopamine is not sufficient already for depressed people to start with, forcing the dopaminergic nerve cells to produce more for their pornographic sessions will further worsen the neurochemical imbalance in the brain. At this point, the brain would likely need pharmacologic intervention to produce the much-needed dopamine, and other neurotransmitters affected such as serotonin, in order to function well.

Pornography and negative mental state

Mental health issues have always been one of the most underestimated conditions, especially in young people. With the strong relationship between neurochemical imbalances with depressive disorder, anything that can wreak havoc on the mental state of an individual can potentially put the patient at risk for depression. One of the most powerful agents for neurochemical imbalances is something that would bathe the brain in pleasure hormones that are stimulated by the wrong factors, this being chronic pornographic consumption. The effects of depressive disorder on the overall psychological function of an individual with pornographic addiction include disturbance in mood, cognitive abilities, psychomotor activities, reminiscing negative memories, speech problems, and even suicidal ideation.

Changing mood and affect. In people who use pornography for a very long time, one may have noticed a change in their general mood, especially around other people. In people who have resorted to porn as a coping mechanism to prior negative childhood history, they are expected to have chronic consumption of porn, enough to rewire the brain and alter their entire personalities. They may have different ways of responding to their friends' conversations, probably using more negative words such as no, not, or never.

Because of the current emotional turmoil that they have whenever they have depressive episodes, they are expected to feel varying levels of sadness, anxiety, guilt, rage, and shame. These feelings reflect how their emotions cannot be regulated, due to the imbalances in neurotransmitters, especially dopamine and serotonin. They may also have a more disapproving non-verbal cue in response to any events or even just in social interactions. For example, a fixed gaze can be observed, implying that their mind is elsewhere, possibly losing focus in a discussion.

Cognition. The capacity of the rational brain to handle, process, and store information is also significantly affected in porn addicts undergoing depressive episodes. This can be manifested as problems in their attention, concentration, and memory.

It can be observed that their attention is affected, manifested in daily social interactions, such as through drifting away in a conversation.

Their concentration will also be compromised, as observed by easily lost focus in activities requiring intensive attention, such as work, or studies. Their memory will also likely be compromised, having an inefficient capacity for holding short-term information, possibly affected by their inattentiveness, and defective long-term memory storage for important information such as study-related teachings, or learned knowledge.

Psychomotor retardation. In addition to emotional and cognitive aspects, the psychomotor function is also affected in the depressed patients. They would seem to manifest with chronic fatigue, though they most likely have spent most of their day in bed. This can be a result of the lack of energy secondary to depressive disorder and fatigue due to overdoing self-induced sexual gratification while using pornography. They can be observed to have much slower general motions, including slow walking, as opposed to the normal pace of an individual. They would also be observed to have lacking facial expressiveness, which reflects the poor affect in depressed individuals, worsened by porn addiction. Most of all, their posture would be more slumped, which is more pronounced than the average slacking posture of people.

These can primarily be observed by family, friends, and colleagues who will notice the subtle changes in the movements and mannerisms of the individual affected. Therefore despite not knowing the person's emotional anguish and history of porn addiction, people can still objectively assume that the person may have depressive episodes due to their change in psychomotor activity.

Ruminative thought processes. In pornography addicts, especially those who have problems with cognition, attention, concentration, and overall emotional regulation, rumination is common. Rumination is a rational behavior of actively thinking and rethinking about past events, especially ones that induce negative emotions. The problem with rumination is that this leads to chaining, where one memory will trigger another memory, which will start an endless cycle of reminiscing about bad moments in one's life. This is highly observable in people who have been using porn consumption as an adaptation to a negative childhood experience.

Speech. In addition to observable signs of changes in non-verbal cues, speech is also significantly affected in depressed people. They may talk much more softly and slowly, with a monotonous voice, spaced with longer and more frequent pauses. They also may seem to lose interest in a conversation, even ones that they are interested in, reflecting the loss of interest in things that they are once passionate about as a result of both depression and porn addiction. They will also be observed to have delayed verbal responses to messages in active conversations, requiring their participation.

Suicidal thoughts. One of the most worrisome signs of depression is suicidal ideation. In people who are addicted to porn and are at risk for low overall self-worth, depression can get them to the point that they will not see value in their life and in their futures. Such was the first individual I've met who confessed to me about this reality. This usually introduces suicidal thoughts to them, thinking that it is the solution to their problem. Having a myriad of complications as pornography addicts, these people would likely have less social support, low self-esteem, and poor motivation to help themselves get through this emotional turmoil. While all of these seem abstract, it is the neurophysiology and neurochemistry of the brain that is the source of these problems manifesting as major depression in porn addicts.

Altogether, these reflect the poor emotional regulation that is rooted in their brain and manifests as observable signs in people who have depression, aggravated by addiction to pornography. These manifestations reflect the significant change in blood flow to the brain regions affected due to depression and are much worsened by chronic dopamine dysregulation secondary to addiction to pornography. The overall gray matter volume will decrease in the region with poor blood flow and thus would result in the poor brain physiology of the affected regions, including cognition, speech, and psychomotor functions. While several of these manifestations seem purely emotional in nature, it is known that depressive disorder patients have a significant difference in brain anatomy upon rewiring of the brain compared to those who have stable mental health.

Management of depression in porn addicts

The primary management to psychosocial and clinical problems related to addiction is to cut the primary root, which in this case is the consumption of pornography. But according to individual cases of chronic porn users, abruptly cutting off porn consumption is highly likely to result in relapse and recurrence in previous addicts struggling to recover from addiction, which is something expected in any journey of recovery. Therefore, the goals of the management have to be very intricate, enough to deal with pornographic addiction as a root cause and a risk factor, as well as manage the depressive signs and symptoms.

The goals of management for people affected with depressive disorder having a history of pornographic addiction include the following:

- **Remission of the depressive signs and symptoms**. This means that there should be resolution of the manifestations of depression, as aggravated by porn addiction.
- **Restoration of the baseline functioning of the affected person**. A primary goal is to revert the person back to their daily normal functioning, without the burden of the complications of depressive disorder and porn addiction.
- **Removal of pornographic consumption as a regular habit.** As one of the possible root causes of depression is the chronic exposure to pornography, it must be stopped. If not, there is a high likelihood of recurrence in the aforementioned problems.

Management plans should ideally include psychotherapy, in addition to the socio-personal support. There are a myriad of psychotherapy options for people who are suspected to have depressive disorders with porn addiction.

Cognitive-behavioral therapy (CBT). As the name implies, it is a combination of cognitive therapy and behavioral therapy which frequently employs patient education, relaxation exercises, therapeutic exposure, coping mechanism training, stress management, or assertiveness training.

The cognitive aspect of the CBT (which can be done separately from the behavioral therapy) includes rationally dissecting the beliefs of the patient. Identifying their suspicions about their condition is vital in this phase in order to correct any distorted and maladaptive beliefs that can interfere with their recovery.

The behavioral aspect for the CBT includes shifting the stimuli of the patient that triggers their problems. Some of the prompts that need to be treated include the triggers to their depressive episodes and any stimuli that raises sexual arousal to start watching pornography.

Interpersonal psychotherapy. This therapy carefully assesses the four internal socio-personal areas that potentially have the problem in the patient, resulting in depression and addiction: **grief over loss, role transitions, interpersonal disputes**, and **interpersonal skill deficits**.

Supportive psychotherapy. This therapy constitutes the improvement of self-esteem, mental functioning, and overall adaptive skills. The self-esteem aspect calls for the assessment of the sense of valuing oneself, through self-regard, self-confidence, and overall self-worth. The psychological functioning is assessed with reality testing, cognitive abilities, and even morals. Adaptive skills tackles the deportment of the person towards their social support system, including their family, close friends, and colleagues. At the end of the process, the person must be able to cope with their internal bereavement enough to gradually cease using pornography to adapt to their negative feelings and experiences, deal with any spontaneous crisis that could lead them to relapse in porn consumption and maintain their overall improvement and dedication to stop porn consumption once and for all.

In addition to these, other psychotherapy can be done as well, such as behavioral activation, family and couples therapy, problem-solving therapy, and psychodynamic psychotherapy. Most importantly, patient education allows them to understand what has been happening to them not only on an emotional level but on a physiological level as well. This orients the person that their manifestations of depressive disorder are indeed caused by their pornographic addiction.

Ineffective defense mechanism for regulation of negative emotions

This may serve as a rabbit hole for pornographic use because some patients justify their dependence on porn as a form of adaptation to the negative mental state they already are in. Meanwhile, they may not be aware that consuming porn does worse to their mental health, soaking their neurons in dopamine and other neurotransmitters that are not meant to be high upon seeing sexually graphic images on the Internet. This affects the regulation of neurotransmitter release, which contributes to a decline in the much-needed neurotransmitters for the regulation of emotions, especially depression. Once pornography becomes the primary stimuli for the release of pleasure hormones, other psychological stimuli would have difficulty increasing the dopamine and serotonin in events that needed emotional regulation, such as any melancholic or anxious event.

While some people justify their use of pornography as a defense mechanism against sad events in their lives through porn-induced pleasure, some people claim to use pornography as a coping mechanism for the loss of physical and sexual relationships. It is no secret that not all individuals have found a stable relationship that would provide them with the warmth and physical connection that humans need. Some of these people self-prescribe the constant use of pornography to substitute physical contact that they may have been craving. This has been thought to be achieved through watching videos of sexual contact, reading stories of real-life encounters by other people, and even watching fan fiction that may or may not happen in real life. As long as there is the simulation of physical contact, it may have a possible target audience that aims to fulfil the longing for a sexual relationship. This may not be effective though, as the audiovisual stimuli brought about by the pornographic materials of today offer different stimuli than an actual physical relationship. It may take time for these people to believe that pornography is actually limiting their potential of being in a relationship.

References:

[1] Willoughby, B. J., Busby, D. M., & Young-Petersen, B. (2018). Understanding Associations between Personal Definitions of Pornography, Using Pornography, and Depression. Sexuality Research and Social Policy. Doi:10.1007/s13178-018-0345-x

[2] Perry, S. L. (2018). Pornography use and depressive symptoms: Examining the role of moral incongruence. Society and Mental Health, 8(3), 195-213.

[3] Borgogna, N. C., Duncan, J., & McDermott, R. C. (2019). Is scrupulosity behind the relationship between problematic pornography viewing and depression, anxiety, and stress? Sexual Addiction & Compulsivity, 1–26. Doi:10.1080/10720162.2019.1567410

Carmona, M. (2022). Is There a Correlation Between Watching Porn & Depression?

Lyness, JM (2022). Unipolar depression in adults: Assessment and diagnosis. Up to Date. Retrieved from: https://www.uptodate.com/contents/unipolar-depression-in-adults-assessment-and-diagnosis

Ch.6

Porn & Narcissism

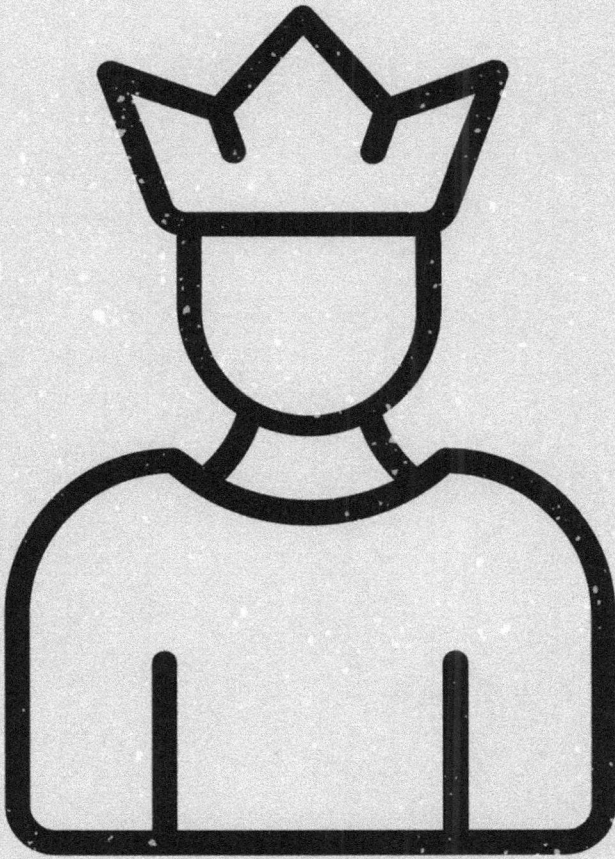

How can pornography contribute to selfishness and narcissistic traits?

Key points discussed in this chapter:

[1] Because pornographic materials depict beyond the realistic sexual experience, such as forms and behaviors, pornography had been an attractive avenue for pleasure in the narcissist. This has been true because of the sexual component of self-admiration, known as sexual narcissism.

[1] In a study, people who have been identified as narcissists through a set of carefully structured assessment exams have been found to be correlated to an increase in the number of hours of using pornography. This denotes that the number of hours spent consuming pornographic content is directly proportional to the narcissistic level of the person.

[1] Several factors have been known to branch out from sexual narcissism: increased sex-seeking behavior, general sexual preoccupation, ownership of sexually explicit materials such as magazines and books, and even sexual aggression.

[1] Sexual narcissists also have been found to have a higher number of sexual partners. Having increased confidence in oneself, the sexual narcissist most likely has a higher amount of social encounters that lead to sexual intercourse.

[2] In studies on adolescents, pornography was viewed as a form of retreat from the transgressions they have in real life, especially as adolescents. Adolescents were described to seek a form of escape from reality and resort to a digital sexual experience where they have an unchallenged omnipotence and feed up their sexually narcissistic behavior.

[3] Findings were more intriguing in women. Narcissism has been found to be associated with women's use of sexual coercion to obtain their individual satisfaction.

[3] Several factors were found to contribute to the conduct of women's use of sexual coercion including poor impulse regulation, emotional modulation, and a heightened sense of sexual desirability.

[3] In women who have been found to have narcissistic personalities, certain approaches have been evaluated with their manner of sexual coercion, including nonverbal sexual persuasion, psychological manipulation and deception, exploitation of the victim while under the influence of a substance, and utilizing physical force or threats.

Introduction:

Martin, a 26-year-old male, is a recently promoted senior engineering manager in a construction firm. While new hires usually gets promotion in a lot longer span of years after onboarding, Martin was promoted while having been on his job for only 3 years. And rumors have it that he got promoted not because of his skills.

Martin was thought to be dating the manager while being an entry-level engineer. Having the guts to date the manager is not a challenge for Martin. After all, he boasts to have gone into relationships with 39 different women in college alone.

"I went out with her, not to get promoted, but just to sleep with her. You know, to add to my *body count*. I was new to the company and I was trying to get a feel of the girls there," Martin confessed as he denies using sex to get ahead of his job. He added that he was just really good at his job, despite his *extracurricular activities*. "For three years since we got this job, my colleagues and I were given the same number of work hours daily, yet I accomplish more. I totally deserved that. The other guys are just jealous because they can't get promoted as fast as I did—even if they were to sleep with our manager."

He invited the team for a celebratory party, where he went on and on about himself. His story focused on three themes—how much he had contributed to every project they had, even just as a junior engineer, how he would rub shoulders with their company executives in anticipation for his future promotions, and how many women he dated and had sex with at different phases of his life. "We had a lot of fun that night. I didn't see any problem, as everybody was laughing and eating well. No one was pitching in their stories, so

I had to keep the conversation going by telling more of mine," he exclaimed.

After the party, he said he left with one of his colleagues and slept with her. "She was laughing extra hard on my stories and kept making eye contact, I thought that was it, that was my cue," he said. When asked if he was worried if his boss that he was dating was aware of it, he said, "Of course not! It was just one night, she doesn't need to know where I always am. Besides, it was purely physical, no attachment at all."

He went home alone, expecting more congratulatory messages via text and social media, but nothing came. He confessed, "It would have been nice if they tagged me on social media with a congratulatory post. After all, I treated them for dinner and gave them a fun night with their future boss—me."

He was referred to the HR regarding inappropriate office behavior and possible sexual harassment. The HR manager, being a psychology graduate and a psychometrician, had extensively evaluated his case and made him take a quick personality test. "I was really surprised—not because I was called to the HR manager's office but because she referred me to a psychologist," he said. "After our discussion, she made me take a quick test that had me realize some of the test questions exactly reflect my attitude, not only towards work, but also towards life as a whole."

Upon further assessment by the psychologist, Martin was found to have a narcissistic personality disorder. Martin confessed to his psychologist that these patterns started during his primary school. His classmate brought an underwear catalogue to school to show to his friends. Envious of their exclusive circle, he brought some magazines of his own and formed another group of boys. "I shared my mags with my other classmates before and we always exchange porn materials. I have this hard drive with gigabytes-worth of pornographic videos that we pass around, which they would have to add to until the memory is full," he confessed. It was his core memory of childhood—whoever had the most porn files that they can share. This translated to whoever had the most sexual experience as early as high school. "I feel completely healthy. I don't think there's any problem with that. Every guy I know watches porn. It's just the way it is," he justified. Despite his extensive pornographic consumption since childhood and the gravity of its effects to him, he never seemed to notice any problem. What he did not know is that his approach to things made him seem to have a superiority complex, making him always look good in every aspect, while unintentionally demeaning the value of the others around him.

Etiology

According to Freud, narcissistic tendencies are correlated to sexual perversions (Sandler, Fonagy & Person, 2012). Though the exact cause of narcissism in pornographic addicts has not been established yet, several studies have shown that biological, hereditary, and psychosocial factors are relevant in these cases.

Neurobiological and genetic causes may have been instrumental to the narcissistic personality that could have been aggravated by any form of addiction, in addition to psychosocial factors. In family and twin studies, personality disorders are found to likely be heritable at 60% of the time, and with 45% concordance in identical twins (Caligor & Petrini, 2022).

From a neurobiological standpoint, brain imaging studies have also found a strong correlation of an impaired empathy in people with narcissistic personality disorders (Caligor & Petrini, 2022). This is one possible reason why narcissistic porn addicts see people as sexual objects more than as humans.

Another relevant cause includes the psychosocial factors that could have instigated the correlation of narcissism and porn addiction.

It is possible that porn addicts use their erotic fantasies and sexual experiences to distract them from feelings of rejection, trauma, or even isolation, which are all aggravated by their narcissistic tendencies (Weiss, 2014). In addition to these, porn addicts may want to cope with emotional tensions, psychological symptoms, and their overall life challenges. As narcissists, these people are more sensitive to rejection and may be prone to being solitary, thus making matters worse. At some point, porn and sex addicts find a way to disconnect from the world, which further isolates them from potential social support, and among these adaptations could be further porn consumption (Weiss, 2014).

Narcissism is also an adaptive mechanism that is potentially caused by feelings of being guilty, inadequate, or unworthy. While some narcissists can achieve real-life success, they maintain a tough front to cover their fragile selves. Successful or not, with an intrapersonal problem like this, they may find a coping mechanism that gives them temporary pleasure, one that they cannot get from approval from others. This is where pornographic addiction sets in.

Sexual narcissism is the strong preoccupation of a person with sex and sex-related concepts (Widman & McNulty, 2010). This includes erotic sensation seeking, strong sexual aggression, and consumption of pornographic content.

Epidemiology

In a study, the degree of narcissism was objectively measured in three different data gathering tools, including the Narcissistic Personality Inventory, the Pathological Narcissistic Inventory, and the Index of Sexual Narcissism. The study found that the higher the number of hours of viewing porn in subjects, the higher degree of their narcissism (Kasper, Short & Milam, 2014). The subjects of the study revealed varying hours of total porn consumption per week, where women claim to take 30 minutes per week watching porn and men take 3 hours, on average. The subjects who admitted to consuming porn scored higher in the scales for testing narcissism levels, consistent with both males and females. Upon extrapolation, porn addicts who consume porn for an estimated 11 to 12 hours at least, may be expected to have much higher degrees of narcissism, though this needs to be confirmed in an actual separate study of its own (Weiss, 2014).

According to several studies, narcissists are more likely to be involved in overly presenting their sexual selves on the Internet, as they are likely to be connected to more virtual friends (Clifton, Turkheimer & Oltmanns, 2009) and actively over-present their positive image to the world (Buffardi, 2011). With greater social connections, sexual narcissists are then expected to have a higher number of sexual partners (Widman & McNulty, 2010).

Pathophysiology

Historically, sexuality has been regarded as a vital part of narcissism, as any narcissistic behavior involved admiration of the sexual aspect of oneself (Levy, Ellison, & Reynoso, 2011).

It was hypothesized that children who had an early severance of caretaker-child relationship could result in failure of the parent to cater to the child's specific needs per developmental period (Caligor & Petrini, 2022).

Through the years of lack of guidance, these deficiencies in parent care would accumulate and the child would be predisposed to having abnormal expectations of and behavior towards other people. This leads to both narcissistic personality as their personality develops through time and porn addiction as their coping mechanism to the lack of love and care as a child.

Upon adulthood, these children with narcissistic personalities are suspected to subliminally seek physical pleasure to validate admiration of them, one that they did not have from their caretakers (Baumeister & Vohs, 2001). With this relevant history, experts also regard narcissistic individuals to be strongly affected by their sexual emotions, which are usually concocted by intense feelings of self-admiration. A good portion of porn addicts, along with sex addicts, were found to be self-centered and self-absorbed, in the sexual aspect and beyond (Weiss, 2014).

This highly reflects how they see themselves as humans. As online pornographic content casts highly idealized persona of men and women, this can be mirrored by narcissists who would like to portray themselves as their best image as well, further increasing their view of themselves as compared to others (Vitz, 2012).

It was also noted that narcissists like to gain as much control of the situations they are in, and the better the control they have on a specific sex object, the more pleasure they obtain from the experience (Akhtar, 2009). Sex object choices can include graphic images, erotic thoughts, or fantasized representations of people. From the eyes of the narcissistic porn addict, they are superior beings, while other humans desirable for them are sex objects that they control.

In light of these findings, scientists have classified these altogether as one concept, bearing both the narcissistic and overtly sexual tendencies of these people, now known as sexual narcissism.

Clinical manifestation

Narcissistic personality disorder is characterized by an outsized sense of self-worth, manifesting with a pervasive pattern of the following tetrad: grandiose sense of **self-importance**, excessive **need for attention and admiration**, having **superficial interpersonal relationships**, and an overall **lack of empathy towards others**. While the development of these features can most likely stem from childhood, these manifestations are expected to be evident upon early adulthood and present in a variety of contexts.

Remember Martin?

He can spend an entire evening talking about himself exaggerating his accomplishments, which shows both the grandiosity of his self-worth and the need for both attention and admiration. His utter disregard of romantic commitment and his ease of sleeping with other women without any strings attached shows how he thrives on superficial social relationships. In addition, the lack of social response, directly or remotely, from his colleagues on his accomplishment shows their relationship with him is superficial as well, that the sense of superficial interpersonal connection is apparently mutual.

When he talks highly about himself, he does so that he inadvertently invalidates the qualities of his other colleagues. Also, he always finds justification of his apathetic actions, such as on why it is okay for him to see other women while building commitment with a partner. These actions show an overall lack of empathy towards others, on Martin's behalf.

Overall, Martin's tendency to be cold and egotistical, while simultaneously needing others' attention and positive regard shows pertinent signs of having a narcissistic personality disorder. This is also backed up by his significant history of pornographic consumption. Martin is a classic case of a sexual narcissist. Narcissistic personality disorder may be identified in people who check at least five characteristics from the following manifestations, especially linking towards their porn and sex addiction (American Psychiatric Association, 2022).

Exaggerated self-importance. A sexual narcissist significantly exaggerates their physical and sexual features, talents, and behaviors, possibly to exude sexual dominance. They expect to be highly recognized as superior among other people, especially those of the same age and sex. The hugely inflated judgments of their own sexual features usually underestimates the characteristics of others, which is known as **devaluation**. The people around them, in turn, receive poorer recognition. For people that have lower emotional quotient surrounding these sexual narcissists, they may be affected and may end up with lower self-worth. On the other hand, other people with stronger personalities may clash with them.

Fantasies of unlimited success. Sexual narcissists are highly convinced that they have unparalleled beauty and exceptional secondary sexual characteristics. When talking about the features that they want to embody, they frequently ruminate about this recognition, especially about their sexual competence. They like hearing and remembering events that acknowledge their features, even if it was just one statement.

Delusion of grandeur. These people also believe that they are unique and deserve to be associated with people who have high-status. Their self-esteem is improved by the idealized persona that they try to embody, which is known as **mirroring**. They usually associate themselves to belong to those people that are well-known, and devalue the characteristics of the people who do not respond to their sense of grandiosity. In more severe instances, they put themselves on a pedestal, besides other well-known people, for example, celebrities, models, or even pornographic actors.

Admiration-requiring. They require excessive attention and admiration, especially regarding their sexual and body features. While they try to present themselves as highly admirable, in terms of their sexual features, their self-esteem is almost invariably fragile. They may feel resentment in people who do not acknowledge their personal features.

Entitlement. These people expect exceptionally favorable treatment. For example they expect people to spread good things about them, especially about their sexual ability, to validate their feelings of superiority.

Exploitative. They will find a way to exploit other people for their own personal good. They take advantage of other people most especially to get sexual advances. This clinical feature makes them conducive to committing acts of sexual violence, such as sexual harassment, non-consensual sexual content, non-consensual sexual intercourse, and sexual exploitation.

Apathy. Sexual narcissists like to take control of their sexual objects for their own gratification. The more control they have, the higher the pleasure they feel. This can be manifested as apathy. Various instances can include apathy to their sexual partners, intention to cheat on their committed partners, and even to gain sexual advances in an otherwise non-consensual fashion. For instance, they may feel intensive apathy to their respective sexual partners, such as after conducting sexual intercourse.

Envy. Another negative aspect of sexual narcissistic personality is the feelings of envy. They may think that other people feel a hidden sense of envy towards them, especially about their sexual features and characteristics. Upon further assessment, sexual narcissists also feel envy towards others, such as those having a stable long-term romantic relationship.

Arrogance. On top of everything, sexual narcissists show haughty behavior that may be off-putting to other people. This can manifest as arrogance, especially emphasizing their pride of their sexuality, secondary sexual features, and overall experiences.

The said clinical and behavioral manifestations reflect that of a narcissistic personality with predisposition towards porn and hypersexuality. In other recognized guidelines, at least three of these are already sufficient to qualify a person under the narcissistic personality disorder. Nevertheless, qualified or not, a person with any of these are guaranteed to have problems with the psychosocial aspect of their lives, and thus requires resolution.

Management and recommendations

It is also important to note that narcissistic personality disorder is among the most difficult to treat conditions, probably since the patient most likely would not see anything wrong, seeing only the good in themselves. It may also be a defect on their pride once they claim to have undergone psychological treatment.

The goals of management in sexual narcissists is to stabilize their condition by treating any acute crises, manage their corresponding pathology, and regain their best possible functionality, despite having the pathology in personality.

Supportive psychotherapy. Conducted by your psychologist, supportive psychotherapy can be a short-term management to treat the person's acute crises such as any narcissistic tendencies, or even as a long-term maintenance therapy, such as to lose porn consumption as a compulsive addiction. The sexual narcissist must be informed that this is a treatment alliance, where the patient themselves must take part in the clinical management of their condition.

The first step in the management of cases of sexual narcissists is awareness about their condition. These people usually do not recognize their faulty personalities, but to treat them, they should know that their approach to things is harmful, not only to other people, but to themselves as well. This can result in the patient obtaining an understanding of their diagnosis, so that they know which attitudes to change. They must know what is right or wrong.

Once awareness is secured, the maladaptive behaviors of the person must be nitpicked to seek the ones that are counterproductive, especially porn consumption. Their clinician, along with the patient, must create a realistic goal on how to gradually change the attitudes that make up their pathological personality. Addictions, such as watching porn, are hard to break, especially if they have been there since childhood. But with active thinking, even a sexual narcissist can stop any maladaptive behavior they have. They can attack the stimulus, changing what they perceive from a once sexual stimulus to a neutral stimulus, thus cancelling out the arousal they feel from it. If that is not possible, they can also modify their actions instead, by doing a different reaction, aside from any sexual advances, towards an otherwise arousing stimulus.

Overall, the sexual narcissist must be guided by their mentor on how to manage destructive actions, to adopt appropriate social skills, and manage negative cognitions. In the long run, porn consumption must be done much less and their behavior towards others must be less constitute of their delusion of grandiose.

References:
[1] Kasper, T. E., Short, M. B., & Milam, A. C. (2015). Narcissism and internet pornography use. Journal of Sex & Marital Therapy, 41, 481–486. doi:10.1080/00926 23X.2014.931313
[2] Wilson, P. J. B. (2018). The porn retreat: Narcissism and adolescence. Psychodynamic Practice, 24(3), 235–244. doi:10.1080/14753634.2018.1494621
[3] Hughes, A., Brewer, G., & Khan, R. (2019). Sexual Coercion by Women: The Influence of Pornography and Narcissistic and Histrionic Personality Disorder Traits. Archives of Sexual Behavior. doi:10.1007/s10508-019-01538-4
American Psychiatric Association. (2022). Personality Disorders. In Diagnostic and statistical manual of mental disorders (5th ed., text rev.). https://doi.org/10.1176/appi. books.9780890425787
Weiss, R. (2014). Narcissism, Porn Use, and Addiction. Psych Central. Retrieved from: https:// psychcentral.com/blog/sex/2014/07/narcissism-porn-use-and-addiction#1

Kasper, T. E., Short, M. B., & Milam, A. C. (2014). Narcissism and Internet Pornography Use. Journal of Sex & Marital Therapy, 41(5), 481–486. doi:10.1080/0092623x.2014.931313

Sandler, J., Fonagy, P., & Person, E. S. (2012). Freud's "On narcissism: An introduction." London: Karnac Books

Levy, K. N., Ellison, W. D., & Reynoso, J. S. (2011). A historical review of narcissism and narcissistic personality. In W.

Campbell, K., & Miller, J.D. (Eds.), The handbook of narcissism and narcissistic personality disorder: Theoretical approaches, empirical findings, and treatments (pp. 3–13). Hoboken, NJ: Wiley

Baumeister, R. F., & Vohs, K. D. (2001). Narcissism as addiction to esteem. Psychological inquiry, 12(4), 206-210.

Widman, L., & McNulty, J. K. (2010). Sexual narcissism and the perpetration of sexual aggression. Archives of Sexual Behavior, 39, 926-939.

Buffardi, L. E. (2011). Narcissism and the World Wide Web. In W. K. Campbell & J. D. Miller (Eds.), The handbook of narcissism and narcissistic personality disorder: Theoretical approaches, empirical findings, and treatments (pp. 371–381). Hoboken, NJ: Wiley.

Clifton, A., Turkheimer, E., & Oltmanns, T. F. (2009). Personality disorder in social networks: Network position as a marker of interpersonal dysfunction. Social Networks, 31, 26–32.

Akhtar, S. (2009). Love, sex, and marriage in the setting of a pathological narcissism. Psychiatric Annals, 39, 185–191.

Barelds, D. H., & Dijkstra, P. (2010). Narcissistic Personality Inventory: Structure of the adapted Dutch version. Scandinavian Journal of Psychology, 51, 132–138.

Caligor, E. & Petrini, M.J. (2022). Narcissistic personality disorder: Epidemiology, pathogenesis, clinical manifestations, course, assessment, and diagnosis. Up to date. Retrieved from: https://www.uptodate.com/contents/narcissistic-personality-disorder-epidemiology-pathogenesis-clinical-manifestations-course-assessment-and-diagnosis

Ch.1

Porn & Shame

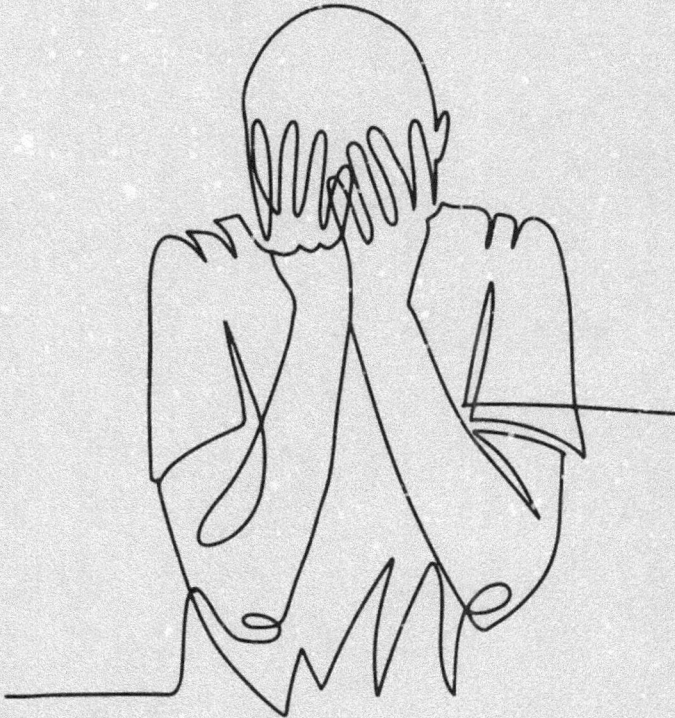

How self-shaming causes several mental crises

Key points discussed in this chapter:
[1] A part of the pathological problem of pornographic addiction is sexual shaming. Although sexual arousal and fantasy is found to be normally part of human nature, this is shamed in people of various cultures, which prompts the person to engage in more discreet and potentially risky sexual behaviors (Kort, 2015).

[1] The normalization of sexual fantasies should be the goal of a healthy society, especially since sexual fantasies were found to have a common theme among people. This can encourage people to express themselves sexually with freedom, rather than engaging in discreet and risky behaviors that predispose them to addiction and other life-threatening risks (Kort, 2015).

[1] If shaming continues, the healthy sexuality of people will be damaged and put them more at risk of pornography addiction (Kort, 2015).

[1] In order to initiate effective management of pornography addiction in people, the history of shame over previous behaviors, sexual fantasies, and any other current sexual activities must be addressed. This frees the person from the mindset of shame and develops the concept of open communication with regard to their sexual needs, which is the first step to healthier sexuality (Kort, 2015).

[2] A significant factor in the conduct of sexual shaming is the childhood household religiosity that convinces the person to think that sexual openness is morally wrong. In domestic settings, children are then forced to conduct sexual experimentation, including using pornographic materials, discreetly, which puts the person at more risk of getting addicted to unsupervised consumption of sexually explicit materials (Volk et al., 2016).

[2] In children, pornographic addiction has been correlated with familial religiosity and moral disapproval, which is built by psychologists as the Religiosity-Moral Disapproval-Perceived Addiction Simple Mediation Model. This predetermines how adults who have pornographic addiction have a likelihood of a history of sexual shaming since childhood (Volk et al., 2016).

[3] Problematic use of porn in men is negatively associated with poorer relationship quality (Stewart, & Szymanski, 2012).

Introduction:

Elle is a Christian girl raised by her mother to be modest and conservative. Though her school friends have been raised in progressive families, she remains committed to her religion. While her friends are going out to eat and watch movies, she stays at home to help her parents with house chores. Until high school, her classmates asked her to join them and hang out with their circles, but she preferred to stay at home with her six siblings to watch TV and play with them. Their regular annual sessions with their guidance counsellors revealed that she has been missing out on a lot of social trends for the age that they need for personality development, such as teen celebrities, pop music, and even cute outfits to wear this summer. "I feel that I am blessed already to have enough of what I need—I live peacefully, I have food to eat, I have a home to warm me in the evenings, and I have a family that I care for," she innocently justified her lifestyle. "I think having friends is optional."

Her guidance counsellor clarified who Elle thinks has been her main influence on how she lives her life. "Did someone teach you to live that way?" he asked.

"My mom said that I am prone to committing sins when I join people who are not committed to their religious faith," Elle responded with no hesitation.

Until the end of high school, she never let her curiosity get in the way of being the obedient Christian girl that she is—until their prom night. Elle was invited to the prom by another Christian boy named, Carlo, from their school. Though they never really hung out before, they saw each other frequently at Church. They only exchanged smiles before, until he approached her to invite her to

92

the prom. "Will you be my prom date?" Carlo asked, to which Elle responded yes. Her mom approved of it since she was friends with Carlo's mom and they regularly chatted regarding church matters.

The prom night was the typical evening for the average high school but nevertheless seemed a confusing night for Elle. Every high school kid there is excited, wearing tux and gowns. It's one night when they can pretend to be grown-ups. Elle thought it would be a dinner and a quickly structured cotillion, but it was more than that.

Throughout the night, she talked to Carlo about the things that she cannot ask her siblings. "Who do you think is the prettiest in our class? What do you like in a girl? Who is your school crush? Have you dated anyone before? How long do you have to hold hands with your boyfriend? How do you know if you can label yourselves boyfriend and girlfriend?" Elle fired a lot of questions which Carlo happily answered without shaming Elle for seemingly being innocent and without any experiences with boys.

As the night went on, they did not notice that the fruit juices that they got from the buffet table were spiked with hard liquor by their classmates. Nothing really happened except Elle's mom noticed that she had an alcoholic flush, with a rosy face, and was further given away by her sluggish speech and her reek of liquor from her breath. Elle's mom thought that Carlo knowingly asked Elle to drink and that Elle was not in her right mind to defend herself. The next morning, Elle insisted that they did not knowingly drink alcohol but Elle's mom did not believe her. She then forbids them from seeing each other again. Elle did not respond well to her mom's reaction.

While she still goes home right after school and does not hang out with any mates at school, she proceeds to lock herself in her room as soon as she gets home. Her prom night may not have been as eventful as other high school kids who proceed to explore with each other, but she has some of her life questions answered—and some left unanswered. Whether these answers given by Carlo are appropriate or not, at least she found someone to talk to. Her mother on the other hand, blocked her away from even opening such conversations at home. At this point, she had not had a chance to explore her sexuality and sexual topics remained to be a mystery to her. "Why is this strictly forbidden? Mom had six children in total, meaning she has done it at least six times," Elle asked herself. "My classmates go on and on at school about their experiences with their boyfriends, and it seems that I'm the only one left behind." Elle took this as a chance to explore.

She started joining online teen blogs to answer her questions on sex and urges. Every answer she was reading led her to nude photos or sexually explicit videos. Elle then started to watch pornographic materials as they seem to be straightforward in showing what she needs to see. This started her three years' worth of pornographic addiction, taking a lot of her time after school up to her years at university. Her family started to notice and her mom snooped on her computer, which revealed her addiction beyond its infancy.

Her mother proceeded to lambast her with hateful words, forcing her to see the guilt that she should be facing. She went on and told her how the rest of the world would perceive her once they knew of her habit of watching porn. In less than an hour of shouting, Elle's mom was able to weigh in on the shame that every Church person, every family friend, and the rest of the world would make her feel. With great embarrassment, Elle's mom referred her to the young pastor of their Church to be blessed and to rid her of the evil spirits that could have caused this. The young pastor realized that the problem is clinical already. She was referred to the psychologist, which is where Elle realized that it had become a problem too. She confessed to feeling ashamed of her habits which have forced her to withdraw from any social circle that offered her company during college. But not only that, she started to feel that she is the problem and not simply her addiction to porn. At the same time, she felt that she missed out a lot in high school already, and learned that she was missing out on college experiences now. She knows that it's a problem, yet she cannot stop the dreaded addiction. When asked about her sexual experiences by peers and potential friends, she could not look them in the eyes and say what satisfies her sexual needs. The shame really weighed on her and she felt helpless.

Reaction of the environment

One of the natural responses of people regarding porn consumption is **sexual shaming** (Kort, 2015). While sexual shaming applies to various activities that are sexual in nature, pornographic consumption is one with the greatest stigma. Sexual shaming is a part of the pathological problem of pornographic addiction contributing to the severity of its manifestations and putting a stigma on those who take part in porn consumption (Kort, 2015). Although sexual arousal and fantasy are found to be normally part of human nature, this is shamed in people of various cultures, which prompts the person to engage in more discreet and potentially risky sexual behaviors.

A significant factor in the conduct of sexual shaming is the childhood **household religiosity** that convinces the person to think that sexual openness is morally wrong (Volk et al., 2016). In some religions, like Islam for instance, moral conducts and religious beliefs and practices are looked at as parallel. However, there are many cultures and other religious groups that are still debating whether pleasuring oneself is immoral or not. In studies involving household religiosity, it was found that they do not discriminate and collectively classify pornography and the act of pleasuring oneself as immoral. They tend to put practices that sets up people to feelings of shame upon learning that sexual indulgence is frowned upon by their religious faith (Volk et al., 2016).

Furthermore, in children, pornographic addiction has been investigated in families that has deep values with familial religiosity and morals, which leads to one of the most powerful responses of the family caretakers and drivers of childhood development, which is disapproval. Psychologists built the Religiosity-Moral Disapproval-Perceived Addiction Simple Mediation Model, which predetermines how adults who have pornographic addiction have a likelihood of a history of sexual shaming since childhood (Volk et al., 2016).

In addition to these, sexual shaming is not confined to the four walls of one's family home. This can also be utilized as a form of retaliation by former romantic partners to their exes, known as **revenge porn**. Revenge porn has also been a problem in the modern times, where former committed partners inadvertently distribute the intimate photos of their exes to others. This results in sexual shaming by society, marking that person as someone who is not worthy of respect. To make matters worse, almost everything on the Internet is forever; once it is published online, it will stay there forever, possibly with multiple copies and with unending uploads. This form of sexual shaming has been found to lead to depression, anxiety, and even suicidal ideations (Amundsen, 2019).

These feelings of shame evolve into grudges, guilt, and eventually despair.

Response to shaming

The fear of sexual shaming precipitates different responses in porn addicts with varying personality types, levels of maturity, and life experiences [1]. Some people who are mature enough to deal with sexual shaming can handle themselves and attack the core problem which is porn addiction. On the other hand, a great number of people will not be mature enough to realize this and will probably fall into the same cycle in an attempt to get out of the addiction. The difference between these people is that level of understanding that is needed here should be objective and unbiased, and where a clear line is drawn between morality and rationality.

It was found in theistic individuals that the higher the degree of scrupulosity, the more severe the shame they feel after every session of using pornography (De Jong & Cook,2021). This roots from their own personal moral disapproval of using pornography.

If shaming continues, the healthy sexuality of people will be damaged and put them more at risk of pornography addiction (Kort, 2015). Pornographic consumption is usually done in closed doors away from the rest of the family, which constitute a more discreet form of pleasuring oneself. People under the spell of porn addiction will think of this as a more practical way of releasing their sexual tension, away from the watchful eyes of the world and thus, away from shame. This emphasizes the value of acceptance of healthy open discussion around sex rather than shaming it and allowing people to resort to porn for learning about the subject and/or to release themselves from sexual urges.

Sex shaming also does something else in the community level. In domestic settings where sex shaming is also rampant, children are forced to conduct sexual experimentation to answer their curiosity, including using pornographic materials, discreetly. This puts the children at more risk of getting addicted to unsupervised consumption of sexually explicit materials, and to the rest of the complications of porn addiction (Volk et al., 2016). This emphasizes the value of sex education in children, rather than letting them explore by themselves with the risk of putting them in the rabbit hole of porn addiction.

In the youth nowadays, they resort to producing alternative accounts in social media besides their actual personal social media account. The alter accounts serve as a way to be anonymous in the World Wide Web, while they partake in digital sexual activities, such as watching sex videos, exchanging nude photos, and even sending provocative messages. This contributes to the tendencies of the youth to engage in high risk sexual activities to release sexual tension. Curiosity fuels the thirst in these youth to seek sexual pleasure, especially for ones who had not experienced it in the rightful age where safe exploration is understandable. Moreover, predisposition to using porn to explore sexual concepts remains one of the longstanding options of these youth in order to sustain their curiosity about sexual ideas, and may one day provide them with inspirations to do high-risk sexual activity themselves.

Porn use results in self-depreciation due to the accumulated shame from chronic use. As it is self-depreciating, it forces the individual to ruminate on his mistakes, and remain unmotivated (Chisholm & Gall, 2015). This takes away the autonomy in the people affected, with them losing their free will to move forward and falling into the endless cycle of porn consumption. This is how porn users end up using more porn, resulting in addiction. This leads to further psychological complications such as depression, anxiety, and stress.

In a study, people, who show disapproval of pornography yet use it themselves, are found to have a tendency to externalize their transgressions to other people, blaming them as the root cause, and that has the potential to ruin relationships (Volk et al., 2019). Putting the blame on others is a convenient way for porn addicts to justify their habits, with much less consequences, for example, a husband may say, because my wife is not doing enough to please me, etc. For the people around them, they should not succumb to these reactions of addicts as they may become vulnerable to the blame and may further help the cycle progress and/or they might believe in the false accusation and develop mental illnesses themselves.

Inherent feelings of shame after porn use

Men consume porn hidden away as they admit to feeling shame after each session of watching sexually explicit videos and masturbating to them (Sniewski & Farvid, 2020). This shame builds over time and ruins one's personality even further. One of the most important values that is affected is autonomy. Porn use erodes autonomy as men experience gradual loss of self-control, which further weakens their fight against addiction (Sniewski & Farvid, 2020). Autonomy also loosens the grip of men in their values and beliefs, which are important foundations of their morals and can be used to empower their self-control and self-discipline. The longer the usage of porn, the more likely autonomy is lost.

In addition to these, female porn users feel even greater shame from a purely female standpoint (Tholander et al., 2022). Based on studies, young women regard porn consumption as "dirty," "disgusting," "hideous," "repugnant," "unnatural," and "vulgar" (Tholander et al., 2022). Porn content usually victimize and objectify women, and women who finds pleasure in these scenes usually feel further shame and disgust after each viewing session. Subjects of the study were found to have highly ambivalent feelings towards pornography, where they feel sexual arousal and inspiration, while also feeling repulsed and shameful (Tholander et al., 2022). Female porn users surmise that they feel the pressure of assuming a supporting role in sex, which hinders their intention of enjoying sex as well for themselves (Tholander et al., 2022). They feel ashamed of speaking out to adjust their sexual relationship to their terms. Inherent shame roots in the personal disapproval of people using pornography (Volk et al., 2019). Acceptance and perception of themselves as addicted to pornography aggravates the shame as it has collectively impacted the individual with every session of porn consumption (Volk et al., 2019).

Management of shame in porn addicts

From the point of view of an individual, the shame should be re-oriented as the reason for them feeling shame is not always right. Justification of the shame would help the person be oriented on what they actually did wrong, which they should feel rightfully guilty of.

In order to initiate effective management of pornography addiction in people, the history of shame over previous behaviors, sexual fantasies, and any other current sexual activities must be addressed. This frees the person from the mindset of shame and develops the concept of open communication with regard to their sexual needs, which is the first step to healthier sexuality (Kort, 2015).

On a larger scale, the normalization of sexual fantasies should be the goal of a healthy society, especially since sexual fantasies were found to have a common theme among people. This can encourage people to express themselves sexually with freedom, rather than engaging in discreet and risky behaviors that prompt them to addiction and other life-threatening risks (Kort, 2015).

Religious beliefs are not necessarily one of the aspects that bring shame to individuals regarding chronic porn consumption. It is the way some people use religions to address such crucial topics that may lead to that shame. For example, spirituality, or developing sincere connection with the Creator has also been studied as a solution to relieve pain and addiction (Chisholm & Gall, 2015). So, it is with the right approach, faith can be used to resolve porn addiction as it still has a sense of focus on rules based on structured beliefs that can be used to curb sexual urges and create a healthier lifestyle. Spirituality-integrated therapy aims to resolve problems in the psychological, emotional, and social well-being of the porn addict (Chisholm & Gall, 2015). With a combination of psychological therapy and self-control, shame can be re-oriented and porn addiction can be resolved.

Spirituality-integrated therapy is one of the methods I have been using to assist clients with addiction to pornography. In my case, however, Islam was the faith utilized.

References:
[1] Kort, J. (2015). Pornography, addiction to ("pro"). The International Encyclopedia of Human Sexuality, 861–1042. doi:10.1002/9781118896877.wbiehs360
[2] Volk, F., Thomas, J., Sosin, L., Jacob, V., & Moen, C. (2016). Religiosity, developmental context, and sexual shame in pornography users: A serial mediation model. Sexual Addiction & Compulsivity, 23(2-3), 244-259.
[3] Simonyi-Gindele, C., Wilson, C., Kuglin, D., Donevan, E., Cole, J., Palmer, J., ... & Snooks, S. How Shame Perpetuates Porn Addiction.
Stewart, D. N., & Szymanski, D. M. (2012). Young Adult Women's Reports of Their Male Romantic Partner's Pornography Use as a Correlate of Their Self-Esteem, Relationship Quality, and Sexual Satisfaction. Sex Roles, 67(5-6), 257–271. doi:10.1007/s11199-012-0164-0
Tholander, M., Johansson, S., Thunell, K., & Dahlström, Ö. (2022). Traces of pornography: Shame, scripted action, and agency in narratives of young Swedish women. Sexuality & Culture, 26(5), 1819-1839.

Sniewski, L., & Farvid, P. (2020). Hidden in shame: Heterosexual men's experiences of self-perceived problematic pornography use. Psychology of Men & Masculinities, 21(2), 201.

Chisholm, M., & Gall, T. L. (2015). Shame and the X-rated Addiction: The Role of Spirituality in Treating Male Pornography Addiction. Sexual Addiction & Compulsivity, 22(4), 259–272. doi:10.1080/10720162.2015.1066279

https://sci-hub.ru/10.1080/10720162.2015.1066279

De Jong, D. C., & Cook, C. (2021). Roles of Religiosity, Obsessive–Compulsive Symptoms, Scrupulosity, and Shame in Self-Perceived Pornography Addiction: A Preregistered Study. Archives of Sexual Behavior, 50(2), 695–709. doi:10.1007/s10508-020-01878-6

Volk, F., Floyd, C. G., Bohannon, K. E., Cole, S. M., McNichol, K. M., Schott, E. A., & Williams, Z. D. (2019). The moderating role of the tendency to blame others in the development of perceived addiction, shame, and depression in pornography users. Sexual Addiction & Compulsivity, 26(3-4), 239-261.

ibid., 1–23. doi:10.1080/10720162.2019.1670301

Amundsen, R. (2019). Cruel Intentions and Social Conventions: Locating the Shame in Revenge Porn. Gender Hate Online, 131–148. doi:10.1007/978-3-319-96226-9_7

Ch.8

Porn & Tolerance

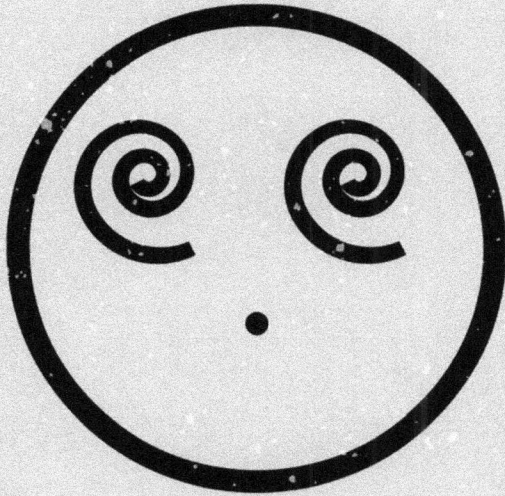

How a porn tolerance trait might cause a person to dislike themselves

Key points discussed in this chapter:

[1] As studies found, heterosexual men are found to compose most of the people afflicted by pornography addiction (Sniewski, & Farvid, 2020). According to one study, subjects who have pornographic addiction are aware of their problem which cannot be controlled due to impulse behaviors. Overall, this leads to tolerance and self-shame.

[2] Tolerance refers to the gradual increase in the required use of pornography through time, in order to achieve a similar level of gratification. (Bőthe et al., 2020).

[2] Tolerance indicates high engagement in an activity and one necessarily pathologic. This may indicate the possibility of treatment in people with tolerance, but the risk of the people undergoing conflict, withdrawal, and relapse symptoms after an attempt to stop porn use.

[3] In addition to these points, pornography contains highly degrading and sexist, and sometimes abusive, content which propagates tolerance to these maltreatment to the subjects of the porn material (Longino, 2018). In the long run, this can translate to societal oppression and demeaning the freedom of the subjects of porn, especially women and children in heterosexual porn materials.

[4] In a book, men's tolerance to sexual violence was discussed to be aggravated by higher rates of porn consumption (Flood, 2010).

[4] In addition to sexual violence, female nymphomania is promoted by pornographic materials in their male audiences which increases the dependence of men, especially the young male audience, on porn for sexual gratification (Flood, 2010).

[4] Porn also sends the unorthodox male sexual prowess which shifts the power dynamics in their sexual practices and relations.

Introduction:

Pornographic addicts usually do not consume porn without knowing the bad effects of this in the individual, at least in the long run of their practice. In fact, porn consumers usually feel shame every time they finish watching porn content and satisfying themselves with it, meaning that they are aware of their wrongdoing. Shame itself roots in their own personal moral disapproval of using pornography as we mentioned in the previous chapter, yet they admit to using pornography regularly (De Jong & Cook, 2021). This is where the concept of each addict's tolerance to using porn comes in.

Nevertheless, they are not safe from the shame that they can feel every session (De Jong & Cook, 2021). Their scrupulosity does not exempt them from the temptation of boosting their dopamine through porn use.

In a study on problematic pornography use, tolerance was previously theorized as a peripheral symptom, being described once as a symptom of high-frequency porn users, but not necessarily the problematic one. The research however proved that tolerance played a more central role in the pathologic consumption of pornography, in both cohorts of people who sought treatment for porn addiction and those who did not (Bőthe et al., 2020). Tolerance is what bridges one-time use of porn to regular porn consumption. It allows the person to consume porn despite being aware of its consequences and the negative message it sends. What forges tolerance into the individual's system are pornographic binges.

The study identified that the so-called pornographic binges, i.e., the repeated use of pornography per day with a higher number of hours per session and/or a higher number of sessions per day, are instrumental to the development of tolerance to porn content (Bőthe et al., 2020). The repeated activity brings about the sense of permission to oneself that you can knowingly consume porn without any direct observable consequences. What porn addicts do not know is that while they are actively tolerating the porn consumption activity, they will gradually manifest guilt and shame from the inside after. But again, this is the behavioral pathology of tolerance: a porn addict will still carry out the activity anyway without the feel or the need of quitting.

Porn addiction changes the perspective of people as well, no matter how scrupulous they are. Tolerance of watching porn allows the individual to do so, despite having contradictory personal traits and values.

In an effort to salvage themselves from the blame, some porn addicts hold other people accountable for their harmful activity. Despite making the decision of consuming porn themselves, hypocrisy or hypocrisy traits rather, set in and could either be defended by denial or pointing them to others. People who intend to hide this habit of theirs in the public usually and unfortunately occur in religious circles, people of faith, or even people who have a strong sense of scrupulosity.

People at risk for tolerance and self-hatred

Tolerating pornographic consumption while knowing that it is wrong serves as a contradiction to the values of respected people in society. But because the pathology of pornographic addiction does not discriminate whether you are a person of high position in society or just an average Joe, chronic use of porn and even sex addiction is usually the dirty secret of respected people.

- **People who hold highly respected positions in society.** People who are in highly respected positions, such the Church goers, practicing Muslims, in politics, or in the educational sector, serve to have limitations in their room for sexual release, due to the sensitivity of these issues in their status. These people include teachers, religious leaders, etc.

- **People who hold higher legal positions and political authority.** In addition to the pressure that their jobs put on them, public servants are inadvertently required by society to be respected enough which limits their capacity for sexual expression. For example, a state prosecutor in the US claimed to be a porn addict to justify his sexually deviant activities, which whether true or not, are found to be incriminating in society's eyes.

- **Professionals consistently exposed to traumatic events.** Field professionals who brave the elements of a dangerous environment and circumstances, such as a war field, scenes with crimes in progress, or traumatic accidents are exposed to heavy physical and emotional stress. Policemen, soldiers, and firefighters are occupations who are at high risk for psychological conditions such as post-traumatic stress disorder and addiction.

- **People who are devoutly religious and with high positions in their religious establishments.** People who abide by religious faith usually have high degrees of scrupulosity and have limited means of expressing their sexuality. This is probably why there are case reports of inappropriate sexual conduct among some religious groups as the restrictions take a toll on their healthy sexual lives.

- **People who are aware of the scientific consequences of porn use.** People who have studied the effects of porn consumption, not only psychologically but also clinically, must have protected themselves from porn addiction—except that addiction does not pick and choose victims. Despite knowing its consequences, porn addiction can still set in, given the circumstances.

The problem with these people who serve to have a high tolerance for porn use is that the longer they hide it in their lives, it can bubble up as worst manifestations, such as physical harm, sexual violence, and even pedophilia.

Harmful effects of tolerance to porn use

From the start, a normal porn user would have watched porn out of curiosity, to belong to their peers, or for sexual satisfaction. Making it into a habit while being aware of any problems it may bring is where tolerance comes in, imprinting the habit into one's lifestyle as acceptable. This has neurological, psychological, and sociological effects on the person.

From a neurologic standpoint, chronic pornography use results in porn tolerance, where the user gets used to the sexual subject and gets less arousal from it from continuous use, thus pushing them to search for more porn subjects. Tolerance was suggested by researchers to cause the reduction of brain volume and gray matter mass, due to desensitization (De Sousa & Lodha, 2017). As an actual manifestation, the person who frequently subjects themselves to a regular stimulus would numb their brain by requiring more dopamine to find sexual satisfaction from that specific stimulus. When this point is reached, the brain would seek more of that stimulus in order to get gratification. This is the phenomenon of **tolerance** in addiction. At this moment, porn addicts have at least two options: they would have to receive the stimuli longer and work harder to reach their climax, or they would have to find a different sexual subject. This brings in the psychological pathology that this neurochemical dysregulation had induced.

From a psychological standpoint, this translates to their behavioral and perceptive state. Achieving tolerance propagates the consumption of porn further by putting the user in an unescapable loop of porn use, where when they get used to one sex object, they can either watch more of it or they can just search for more, in place. In response, this alters the sexual taste of the individual which can reflect on their preference for a sexual partner and any sexual activities they would like to do in the near future. Imagine having a great number of porn addicts in one community, especially in the vulnerable population such as adolescents and high-stress occupations. This connects the neuropsychological standpoints to the societal problems porn tolerance brings.

From a sociological standpoint, the harms of porn tolerance do not end with the user. The content from pornographic materials is promoted strongly on the Internet. While the motivation for this is probably for profits of the websites, they are also inadvertently promoting whatever theme the porn contents contain. Pornography contains highly degrading and sexist, and sometimes abusive, content which propagates tolerance to maltreatment of the subjects of the porn material (Longino, 2018). In the long run, this can translate to societal oppression and demeaning the freedom of the subjects of porn, especially women and children in heterosexual porn materials.

This brings to mind an old friend of mine who, back in the day, attempted to rape a girl while he was on the grounds of her school and was consequently sentenced to some time in jail for his crime. We were all startled at what he did, and he later admitted to me that he was addicted to these types of pornographic acts when he was younger.

Another societal implication of this is the unequal treatment of genders in porn content. Female nymphomania is promoted by pornographic materials to their male audiences which increases dependence of men, especially the young male audience, on porn for sexual gratification (Flood, 2010). This also gives a wrong impression to the public that all women demand overly high amounts of sexual satisfaction, enough to resort to unorthodox sexual practices such as voyeurism, sexual assault, and non-consensual sex, just like how they depict it in porn materials.

Moreover, men who regularly consume porn actually develop a tolerance for these sexually inappropriate practices. In the book *Everyday Pornography*, men's tolerance to sexual violence was discussed to be aggravated by much higher rates of porn consumption (Flood, 2010). Tolerance of sexual violence can potentially branch to the risk of doing illegal sexual offences thereby inducing actual harm to other people.

In addition to sexual violence, porn also promotes the unorthodox male sexual prowess which shifts the power dynamics in their sexual practices and relations (Flood, 2010). This can result in problems with sexual gratification whenever the porn addict already engages in actual human sexual activity. Much worse, this can increase the expectations of men in a sexual relationship, demanding more from their female partners, which can result in much less sexual satisfaction on behalf of the women.

Furthermore, with an increasing number of porn consumption in today's men, it has become instrumental in the hastened sexual maturity of boys and contributes to their interpersonal peer culture and socio-sexual relations. The environmental aspects that introduce the concept of sex to young people expose them to highly mature and aggressive content, that the young mind is not yet ready to even process. This is one of the reasons for the officially established age of legal sexual consent, to ensure that no one under the prescribed age would engage in sexual activity that may be too much to handle for a child's mind. But is there anyone to monitor that?

Manifestations of porn addiction in people who reached tolerance

Porn addiction entails the frequent use of pornography, whether with or without awareness of its complications to one's health and well-being. The main characteristic of people who are tolerant to the usage of porn as compared to those who are not, is that they actively consume porn, despite being against it. This ironic logic of these people denotes another aspect that needs to be resolved. Though awareness is ideal, tolerance of doing something wrong shows a fault in the character of these people. The following are the behavioral and socio-personal manifestations of porn addicts who have maintained tolerance in the act.

Promoting against porn, despite actively using it. Telling people that porn consumption is wrong despite doing it themselves emphasizes that the individuals themselves know the right from the wrong but somehow do not abide by their own principles. Having an active opinion against porn does not always mean that they get to abide by their own words themselves. While this shows distaste from the perspective of other people, if one is looking into resolving this, someone must inform them that their awareness must translate into actions.

Feelings of shame and guilt after each porn session. Because they know that consuming porn is bad for their general well-being, they still feel guilty every time they use porn. Depending on the timeline of usage of porn in these people, they may have varying degrees of shame upon using. Porn audiences range from the newbie porn user who is just starting to fall into the cycle of porn addiction to long-term porn consumers who have learned to live with the shame of everyday porn use. Whatever their timeline is, they are expected to be ashamed at some point, which reflects their knowledge that the action is wrong.

Shaming people for consuming porn despite usage. Having the guts to shame another person whilst using porn is one of the extreme manifestations of tolerance. This is when a person has accepted that they are doing it and they know that they would not receive any consequences because they can lie about using it. This action entails dishonesty, redirecting the topic to other people on how they use porn, making sure that they do not reveal of their own addiction.

Being biased in their opinions about porn. Being against it in general, but being actively accepting of it when talking about porn usage with close friends shows a degree of inconsistency in their values and stand against porn. These people want to show the general public that they too are against the act of porn consumption, yet they openly practice it in real life and it is probably known to their close friends or even spouses.

Lying about using porn and being defensive about it. Tolerant people also have a tendency of being defensive about using porn. This reveals the aspect of denial, which is their psychological defensive mechanism against an action that they do not want to be known to other people. The shame of using pornography is their motivation to lie about it. It has become an intrinsic mechanism to defend their good perspective of themselves, hoping that others will remain to see that.

Management of porn addiction in people who reached tolerance

Tolerance is the point where the porn addict has accepted that despite their knowledge that porn consumption is wrong, they still continue to partake in it. The knowledge of the act and its respective consequences is not enough for them to stop.

Tolerance indicates high engagement of an activity and one necessarily pathologic. This may indicate the possibility of treatment in people with tolerance, but there is a risk of the people undergoing conflict, withdrawal, and relapse symptoms after an attempt to stop porn use. People who are identified to have greater tolerance of porn may be at a higher risk (Bőthe et al., 2020).

Action. Awareness is usually the first step in managing addiction. But in people who have developed tolerance, they continue to take part in porn consumption despite awareness. They have reached the point of acceptance of being a porn addict while knowingly suffering the consequences. Therefore, the first step for these people is developing a plan of action. With the knowledge of the addiction itself, it would be a natural next step to figure out the specific aspects of their addiction: where does their need for watching porn come from? These people may be deprived of sex from their committed partners, or they may have limitations in sexual activity secondary to religious rules, etc. These require specific internal actions that can solve their dire position of being porn addicts while knowing that it is wrong.

Break down. Upon completing the plan of action, one must observe the results. Are they responding well to their plan of action? Do they comply with abstinence? If not, why do they keep failing? They can ask these questions and readjust their approach. They must break down the actions that they can and cannot do, and the ones that they can sustain. They must also break down where and when they consume porn.

Control. At this point, the porn addict must have determined the factors that allow them to consume porn, and the reasons why they wanted to watch porn in the first place. The goal is to make the action sustainable. The next step then is to control, both themselves and their environment.

Self-control means taking actions that help oneself not only quit the consumption of porn, but also to engage in other actions that will bring about more benefits to one's life. Utilizing alarms to allow them to stick to a schedule and prevent them from allotting time for porn consumption can be useful.

Controlling the environment means that one should optimize the environment they live in and make it work for them in their battle against porn addiction. Their environments must become conducive to whatever good they want to achieve in life. If they frequently access porn on their desktop while alone in their bedrooms, they can move their desktop to a common room in the house. If their porn consumption is promoted by using their phone in the bathroom, then make your bathrooms a no-phone zone. Do you consume Internet pornography in the middle of the night? Schedule your Internet connection to be turned off at night, when you should be sleeping instead of being online, whether doing porn or not.

Discipline. After controlling the self and the environment, maintaining these as habits is the difficult part. Long-term solutions entail maintaining healthy habits that stick to the end. It may be easy to stumble upon old unhealthy habits, especially when you are dealing with neurochemical imbalances, which defies the most rational minds.

Any imbalances in dopamine, serotonin, and norepinephrine, can all derail the sharpest minds of their plans. So fix your mind on getting things done, day in and day out. Getting an accountability partner is effective. Looking for a community with the same goals also works. Whatever the case is, discipline is to do what you know is right, whether you like it or not.

References:
[1] Sniewski, L., & Farvid, P. (2020). Hidden in shame: Heterosexual men's experiences of self-perceived problematic pornography use. Psychology of Men & Masculinities, 21(2), 201.
De Jong, D. C., & Cook, C. (2021). Roles of Religiosity, Obsessive–Compulsive Symptoms, Scrupulosity, and Shame in Self-Perceived Pornography Addiction: A Preregistered Study. Archives of Sexual Behavior, 50(2), 695–709. doi:10.1007/s10508-020-01878-6
[2] Bőthe, B., Lonza, A., Štulhofer, A., & Demetrovics, Z. (2020). Symptoms of problematic pornography use in a sample of treatment considering and treatment non-considering men: A network approach. The Journal of Sexual Medicine, 17(10), 2016-2028.
[3] Longino, H. E. (2018). Pornography, oppression, and freedom: A closer look. In Living with Contradictions (pp. 154-161). Routledge.
[4] Flood, M. (2010). Young men using pornography. In Everyday pornography (pp. 176-190). Routledge.
[5] Kalman, T. P. (2008). Clinical Encounters with Internet Pornography. The Journal of the American Academy of Psychoanalysis and Dynamic Psychiatry, 36(4), 593–618. doi:10.1521/jaap.2008.36.4.593
De Sousa, A., & Lodha, P. (2017). Neurobiology of Pornography Addiction–A clinical review. Telangana journal of psychiatry, 3(2), 66.

Ch.1

Porn & mood swinging

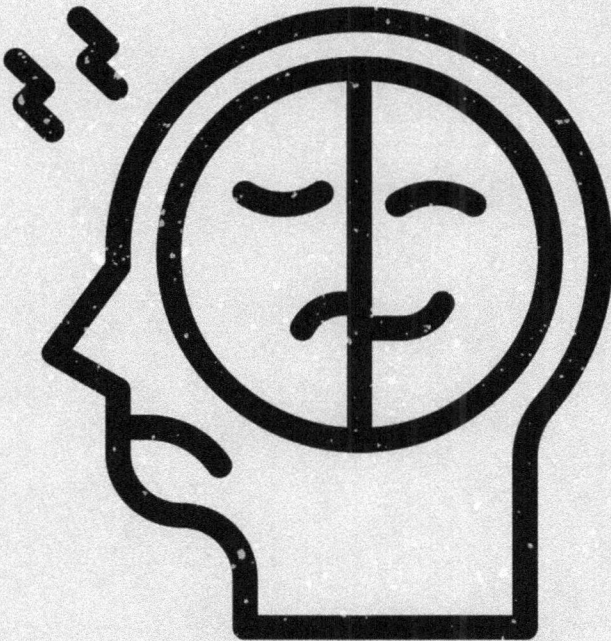

Porn and its potential to distract from life's essentials and necessities.

Key points discussed in this chapter:

*[1] In a study, pornographic addiction is technically called **Internet-pornography-viewing disorder (IPD)** under internet-use disorder, which is being studied on its effects on mood alteration depending on the severity of Internet-use addiction. With the added burden of internet addiction, the changes in neurotransmitter balance induced by pornographic consumption result in a much worse condition in a person with regular exposure to pornography.*

[1] The Internet-pornography-viewing disorder has been found to negatively impact calmness, energy, and an overall good mood in the individual. In addition to this, the disorder was found to have a bad effect on emotional avoidance, excitation seeking, and the overall feeling of sexual arousal, all of which contributes to the mood of the person.

[2] In another study, the negative mood brought about by exposure to sexually explicit images has been found to affect certain performance tasks in the subjects.

[3] Problematic porn users were investigated to identify symptoms of their condition, which include the motivation of porn use for mood modification, i.e., to decrease negative mood, such as sadness and stress. Other studies investigate mood modification as a form of euphoria, i.e., a positive reinforcement through inducing pleasure after doing a specific set of behavior (Bőth, et al., 2020).

[3] In the study, the subjects who actively sought treatment for problematic pornography use were found to have mood modification as their central symptom. This could emphasize that the motivation of people who have earlier acceptance of their condition and are proactive enough to resolve it use pornography for mood modification, i.e., to feel good in place of an existing negative emotion.

Introduction

Mood modification is characterized as a disruption in neurocognitive, psychologic, and socio-personal functions, significantly affecting daily interpersonal, intrapersonal, and professional functioning (Suppress, 2023). Disturbance in neuropsychologic aspects involves regular mood changes out of the ordinary for the affected person, in

119

addition to changes in levels of energy, a heightened rate of activity, changes in sleep requirement, a decline in executive function, and overall modification in behavior (Suppress, 2023). If symptoms worsen, episodes of manic, hypomanic, and major depressive manifestations can be tell-tale signs of bipolar disorder, which may require professional guidance.

Mood changes were previously hypothesized to be a peripheral symptom of porn addiction, as compared to more pressing symptoms. However, based on a study, the Problematic Pornography Consumption Scale was used to check the level of mood modification in people who admit to having porn addiction and are open to or are undergoing treatment (Bothe et al., 2020). The study found that mood modification is a central manifestation of porn addiction, and thus requires more attention.

If not treated, the mood problems in porn addicts can possibly progress to alternating mood syndromes, which further puts the individual in more psychological comorbidities. This syndrome is morbid enough to initiate high-risk activities in the affected individuals, or worse, suicidal ideations.

This section discusses the results of mood disturbances in porn addicts, the pathophysiology of mood changes in porn addicts, manifestations of mania and hypomania and their relation to porn addiction, management of mood changes in porn addicts, and mood modifications in porn withdrawal.

Results of mood disturbances in porn addicts

Mood disturbances significantly affect the general brain function including neurologic, psychologic, and socio-personal functions, because of the effect of mood swings in neurophysiology (Suppress, 2023).

Neurocognitive function. While general intelligence is mildly affected by any disturbance in mood, other cognitive functions can be significantly affected. These include focus, verbal memory, executive function, and rate of processing information.

Focus, being a valuable asset in today's society, is one of the domains that is affected by mood disturbances in porn addicts. For people with mood disturbances, it is usually difficult to get a hold of their attention for a longer time due to their predisposition to shift their focus to less relevant stimuli. In combination with the other symptoms, loss of focus can be an important effect of mood changes.

Verbal memory, or the capacity to receive, process, and store information that is disseminated verbally, can be affected by these mood changes as well. A porn addict can manifest with regular mood swings and gradually observe that they have to repeatedly be communicated with regarding matters that have been discussed already. To objectively test the affected person, several tests can be used such as prescribed word lists, story recall, logical memory, and testing retention of paired words in sequences (Suppress, 2023).

Cognitive function, especially the capacity for executive functioning, is one of the most relevant domains affected by mood disturbances in people. The capability of planning, concept or set shifting, and response inhibition are, after all, a huge part of what sets humans apart from other organisms. Once these are affected, the capacity of the individual to function well in the real world, especially in the professional setting, will be impacted.

The rate of processing information is also gravely decreased in people with mood disturbance. This may be correlated with the loss of focus and verbal memory of the individual, which limits their capacity to perceive the much-needed information for processing. With a decreased information processing speed, porn addicts may have much less efficiency in their daily functioning.

Social and interpersonal skills. One of the most valuable social skills that reflects higher emotional quotients includes the capacity to recognize the thoughts of another human being, which is unfortunately decreased in people with mood disturbance. This skill is described by the "theory of mind" where an individual can infer the likely thoughts, values, and intentions of other people, as well as of themselves. The ability to practice this opens a lot of possibilities for making social connections, which in porn addicts manifesting with mood disturbance, would be difficult to do.

In addition to this, the capacity to predict standard human emotions such as joy, despair, terror, rage, and even surprise in other people is impaired as well. In the real world, this skill is usually executed by the ability of people to recognize the facial expression of another person, in addition to emotional processing. Altogether this will be interpreted by the mind as a definitive emotion, which allows the individual to react appropriately to the ongoing feelings of another person. In porn addicts feeling mood changes, this may be really difficult.

An important link between the neurocognitive and social skills of an individual is the capacity to make practical decisions appropriate for a specific event. This can be done by weighing the pros and cons of the particular decision, and the corresponding rewards and punishments. If the person has mood disturbances, these decisions may seriously be compromised based on their ongoing mood.

Neurocognitive and social skills are important backbones of the human as a social individual. Without these skills, it may be difficult to comply with social norms, be accepted by their peers, and ultimately belong to society at large.

Mood pathology in porn addicts

Porn addiction brings about a cascade of neurophysiological effects that impairs the psychological functioning of an individual (Suppress, 2023). The chronic boost of dopamine upon utilization of pornographic materials for sexual gratification can take its toll on neurochemistry (Kamaruddin, Rahman & Handiyani, 2018). The normal neurotransmitter balance in normal situations will be derailed, often when it is needed most, such as in situations requiring emotional regulation, cognitive function, and overall neuropsychologic normalcy (Kamaruddin, Rahman & Handiyani, 2018). Though few studies focus on the effect of porn addiction on mood modification, the usual pathology of mood disturbance can be correlated to this behavioral addiction. The following are the pathology of mood disturbance in people, which are potentially more pronounced in porn addicts.

Prodrome. On top of mood manifestations, non-mood prodromal symptomatology are indicative of mood disturbance. Expected in porn addicts as an effect of neurochemical disequilibrium, affected individuals are expected to manifest with increased mood lability, more commonly known to lay people as mood swings. This can include elevated mood, manifesting with hyperactivity and agitation, which in extension can eventually progress with irritability and aggressiveness. On the other hand, certain episodes may manifest with the complete opposite mood, manifesting as depression, anxiety, and even panic.

123

In individuals who chronically manifest with these prodromal symptoms, it can induce sleep disturbance. Effects to sleep are variable, as some people may manifest with decreased needs for sleep due to unexplainable reasons, while others, especially those with depressed moods, can manifest with a complete lack of sleep or be at risk of oversleeping.

In much worse cases, disruptive behaviors are expected which can eventually be diagnosed as other disorders such as conduct disorder. Worse still, if the patients are left untreated, they could be left with psychotic experiences, such as delusions or hallucinations, as early as their prodromal period.

Mania. If these prodromal symptoms persist, mania can be expected from the affected individuals. Manic episodes are characterized by clinically significant modifications in mood out of the normal personality of the individual, as well as changes in vitality, actions, conduct, rest, and thinking capacity.

Hypomania. On a similar note as mania, hypomanic episodes are also characterized by changes in vitality, actions, conduct, rest, and thinking capacity, but have much less severity. If left unmanaged, this can result in psychological comorbidities.

Major depression. Once the mood disturbances are accompanied by depressive episodes, the person should already be assessed for other mental health problems. Bipolar disorder is usually characterized by major depressive episodes on top of manic and hypomanic episodes. The manifestations of major depression have their own complications and can make matters much worse for the porn addict.

Psychosis. In severe cases, the manic, hypomanic, and major depressive episodes may be aggravated by clinically significant psychotic symptoms such as delusions, hallucinations, and disorganized train of thought and conduct.

The evolution of mood disturbances in porn consumers is initiated and aggravated collectively by the neurochemical disturbances, psychological manifestations, and overall sociological implications of porn addiction. These sets of pathologies are highly technical for individuals to determine by themselves. Some clinical manifestations of these mood labilities may come in handy for taking note if a porn consumer is already indicated for further assessment by a professional.

Mania and hypomania in porn addicts

Mood disturbance is more than meets the eye. Mood entails varying presentations, depending on the specific instance. The symptomatology of mania and hypomania in porn and sex addicts, guided by the criteria for bipolar disorder as defined by the American Psychiatric Association (2022) presents a more objective look at these behavioral manifestations. Given that mood modification in porn addiction is not yet well-studied, these clinical manifestations are a good start in identifying mood disturbance in porn addicts and possibly sex addicts as well.

Irritable or expansive mood. People with mood disturbances can have certain episodes of expansive mood that can last for several days. With these intense periods of time, they may require high levels of sexually arousing activities. These manifest as unexplainably expansive moods or high degrees of irritability that usually cannot be resolved by non-clinical means.

Persistently high energy. Certain episodes grant affected people unexplainable high energies, which cannot usually be reciprocated by normal people. One of the expected results of this is to engage in activities that will expend this energy and with poorer decision-making skills, these people may be at risk for sexually inappropriate activities including sexual infidelity or sexual encounters.

Observed changes in mood by other people. Mood changes are not usually observed firsthand by the individual affected. Therefore, clinicians may be dependent on the observations of other people regarding the changes in the mood of the affected person. Disturbance in mood as seen by other individuals is a much more reliable way of assessing if the individual has any significant changes in their way of expressing oneself or in engaging in different activities that they are not used to.

Additional mood-altering symptoms. During episodes of mood disturbance, three or more symptoms can be expected to manifest.

1. **Inflated self-esteem, potentially promoting their sexuality.** The elevated mood in the affected person lifts their spirits and inflates their self-esteem, which gives them unearned confidence to do activities that they usually don't do. This makes for a worse manifestation if the person engages in bad decisions.

2. **Decreased need for rest and sleep.** An elevated mood also improves the energy of these individuals, which manifests as a decreased need for rest. While completely unexplainable by other conditions, the boost in energy is usually translated to activities that are unwise in very specific situations. For example, people with high energy and inflated self-esteem are likely to engage in inappropriate sexual activity, such as infidelity.

3. **Talkativeness.** The person with an elevated mood adopts loquacious behavior, even if they are not usually talkative in normal situations. They may feel an unexplained internal pressure to keep talking, which may or may not be pleasant to their peers. With the other problems in cognition in porn addicts with mood modification, they may say something distasteful out loud.

4. **Flight of ideas, especially sexual in nature.** The person experiences an increased flow of thoughts that are inconsistent and not aligned with the topics currently being discussed. In porn and sex addicts, these ideas are usually sexual in nature. Combined with their talkative nature, people with elevated moods may express inappropriate ideas not aligned with the situation at hand.

5. **Distractibility.** Consistent with the other symptoms, the affected person may have an increased risk of losing focus on an object of attention, usually by irrelevant stimuli. Being distracted constitutes one of the flaws in the cognition of the porn addict, affecting the reception of information and resulting in problems with executive skills.

6. **High desire to achieve any goal-directed activity, usually sexual satisfaction.** With the high energy cooped up in these individuals, they may have the exceptional desire to achieve a specific goal. While this may sound advantageous in a normal instance, it is important to take note that these people usually do not have the correct compass for decision-making and thus may pursue activities that are out of line with their own principles. One aspect that may be relevant here is porn addicts include activities that are sexual in nature, despite it being opposed to their normal persona.

7. **Severe involvement in high-risk activities, including sexual indiscretions.** While in a state of mood disturbance,

the porn addict may not be in the best condition to think well about their actions, before they commit to them. An important example of these high-risk activities is sexual indiscretion and relationship infidelities. Altogether, they end up making bad decisions they would never make if they were not in a state of mood disturbance.

8. **Severe mood disturbances result in problems in one's daily life**. Affected individuals may experience severe mood swings enough to result in a disturbance in daily social and occupational functioning. This may be relevant to relationships and can even affect their professional lives.

9. **Risk-taking behaviors and suicidal ideations.** If these clinical manifestations present with significant impulsive conduct that are out of line with the individual's personality, this may be a more severe form of mood disturbance. In addition to this, suicidal thoughts and behavior may be elicited from the clinical history of the affected individual.

It must be noted that these symptoms should not be related to any exogenous factors that may trigger such disturbance in mood. Episodes should therefore not be attributable to any biochemical or exogenous factors such as illicit drugs, alcohol, or nicotine products.

Psychologic comorbidities in individuals with mood disturbances include major depression. From the other perspective of the manic and hypomanic moods in these individuals, the affected person is at risk for major depressive manifestations, which would further qualify them for bipolar disorders.

Bipolar disorder. This can be diagnosed in affected individuals who are observed to have either of the following manifestations:

manic episodes, as well as high frequency of major depressive and hypomanic episodes, thereby classified as bipolar disorder I; or at least one of the episodes each of hypomanic and major depressive manifestations, without the manic events, thereby classified as bipolar disorder II.

If the symptoms are carefully assessed by psychologists and psychiatrists, bipolar disorder can possibly be diagnosed in these cases. Though fewer studies were tackled regarding this matter, porn addiction symptoms can potentially contribute to the mood swings of an individual, putting them at further risk for having bipolar disorder.

As much as awareness of these clinical manifestations is important when observing your close family and friends, knowledge of these clinical presentations is also important for self-management in a porn addict. But dealing with the mood disturbance itself may not be sufficient to resolve the whole pathology.

Mood swings upon withdrawal from porn

Emotional distraught such as mood disturbance manifesting as stress, anxiety, or even depression, are established manifestations of addiction to any etiologies, including substance and behavioral addictions (Fernandez et al., 2023). As guided by Griffiths' (2005) components model of addiction, the factors assessed to check the condition of a suspected patient with addiction include salience, conflict, withdrawal, tolerance, relapse, and mood modification. Being a vital part of the criteria, mood modification has been used as a measure of how severe the form of addiction affects the individual (Fernandez et al., 2023). Because porn addiction wreaks havoc in the normal neurochemistry of the brain, the mood is one of the normal aspects of the individual that is destabilized once the addiction takes place, more so once the withdrawal is initiated.

Despite the undesirable consequences, withdrawal is an important process to go through when cutting the addiction to porn consumption once and for all (Fernandez et al., 2023). The problem with withdrawal symptoms is that former porn addicts who are attempting to recover, subjectively thought that the manifestations of abstinence are much worse than their observable symptoms while being addicted to porn (Fernandez et al., 2023). This places recovering porn addicts at great risk of relapse, because of their uncomfortable mood manifestations, on top of other withdrawal symptoms.

Management of mood swings in porn addicts

With a combination of pathologies in the neurophysiologic and psychological domains of the individual, mood disturbances may present worse enough to be indicated for clinical management. However, in porn addicts, this may not be as easy as treating the mood pathology. With this in mind, the management goals for co-manifestation of mood disturbance and porn addiction include the following: to stabilize the mood of the affected individual, to prevent the recurrence of the mood pathology and related manifestations, and the overall resolution of porn addiction (Vieta & Colom, 2023). It is important to note that severe manifestations of mood disturbances may call for pharmacotherapeutic interventions, which need to be prescribed by a psychiatrist. For the purpose of this entry, the non-pharmacologic interventions will be focused on.

Group and individual psychoeducation. The objective of psychoeducation is to guide the patient to safely make them aware of their condition, to advise them of their manifestations and the potential management plans, and to encourage them to be proactive in self-management. (Vieta & Colom, 2023). It is important to carefully make the person aware of their manifestations, as they may not be in the right state to receive any negative comments. As difficult as it may be, awareness is the first step to the resolution of mood disturbance and porn addiction, alike. Once aware, this must initiate treatment-seeking behavior that will improve the outcomes of management for the affected person. This will also improve the chance of self-management.

Vigilance on prodromal symptoms and self-management. They must be vigilant in their manifestations, especially in the prodrome, where the symptoms are just starting to take place. These include habits that the person can incorporate into their lives to prevent the worsening of their condition. These will also guide them to actively manage their symptoms, which can greatly improve their treatment outcomes. In addition to this, the person must be carefully educated on self-management. Firstly, giving them hope for change is important, as this encourages them to believe that it is indeed feasible to recover from this problem. As this is also a highly stressful condition for the person, they can be advised to find ways to calm themselves from stress, such as through mindfulness-based stress reduction. Dietary modifications can also improve outcomes, advising them to regulate their carbohydrate and fat intake which can disrupt hormonal balances and can affect mood. Furthermore, exercise is a good way to improve naturally occurring endorphins, which improves mood, on top of improving overall health and wellness (Vieta & Colom, 2023).

Psychotherapies. The prescribed psychotherapies for people with mood disturbances include interpersonal therapy, social rhythm therapy, or control therapy. In addition to these, group psychoeducation, cognitive-behavioral therapy, or family therapy are also recommended for dealing with both mood disturbances and behavioral addiction, such as chronic porn use (Vieta & Colom, 2023).

References:
[1] Laier, C., & Brand, M. (2017). Mood changes after watching pornography on the Internet are linked to tendencies towards Internet-pornography-viewing disorder. Addictive behaviors reports, 5, 9-13.
[2] Markert, C., Baranowski, A. M., Koch, S., Stark, R., & Strahler, J. (2022). The Impact of Negative Mood on Event-Related Potentials When Viewing Pornographic Pictures. Frontiers in Psychology, 12, 673023.
[3] Bőthe, B., Lonza, A., Štulhofer, A., & Demetrovics, Z. (2020). Symptoms of problematic pornography use in a sample of treatment considering and treatment non-considering men: A network approach. The Journal of Sexual Medicine, 17(10), 2016-2028. https://doi.org/10.1016/j.jsxm.2020.05.030
Fernandez, D. P., Kuss, D. J., Justice, L. V., Fernandez, E. F., & Griffiths, M. D. (2023). Effects of a 7-Day Pornography Abstinence Period on Withdrawal-Related Symptoms in Regular Pornography Users: A Randomized Controlled Study. Archives of Sexual Behavior, 1-22.
American Psychiatric Association (2022). Personality Disorders. In Diagnostic and statistical manual of mental disorders (5th ed., text rev.). https://doi.org/10.1176/appi.books.9780890425787
Suppress, T. (2023). Bipolar disorder in adults: Clinical features. Up to Date. Retrieved from: https://www.uptodate.com/contents/bipolar-disorder-in-adults-clinical-feature
Post, R.M. (2023). Bipolar disorder in adults: Choosing maintenance treatment. Up to Date. Retrieved from: https://www.uptodate.com/contents/bipolar-disorder-in-adults-choosing-maintenance-treatment
Vieta, E. & Colom, F. (2023). Bipolar disorder in adults: Psychoeducation and other adjunctive maintenance psychotherapies. Up to Date. Retrieved from: https://www.uptodate.com/contents/bipolar-disorder-in-adults-psychoeducation-and-other-adjunctive-maintenance-psychotherapies
Griffiths, M. (2005). A 'components' model of addiction within a biopsychosocial framework. Journal of Substance use, 10(4), 191-197.
Kamaruddin, N., Rahman, A. W. A., & Handiyani, D. (2018). Pornography addiction detection based on neurophysiological computational approach. Indonesian Journal of Electrical Engineering and Computer Science, 10(1), 138-145.

Porn & emotional detachment

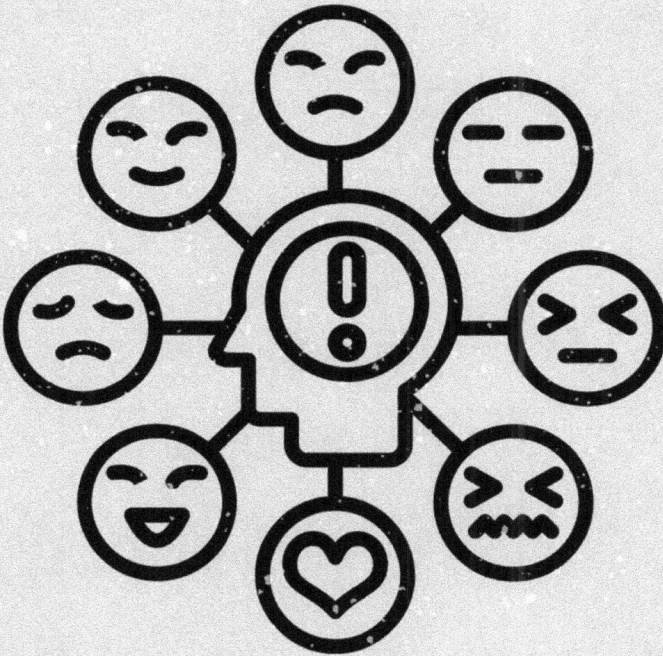

How pornography consumption ruins and alters your feelings for your loved ones

Key points discussed in this chapter:

[1] Relationship status has been a vital factor in the porn-seeking behavior of people. In some cohorts, couples grow colder through time and therefore have much lesser physical contact and sexual activity, which can result in porn-seeking behavior in some people (Brown et al., 2017).

[1] Divorced people have a 25% higher chance of seeking pornographic material than single people. This is probably to supplement the loss of physical contact and sexual activity with their previous betrothed, which results in pornographic-seeking behavior (Brown et al., 2017).

[1] Once married, people have been found to consume 20% less pornography (Brown et al., 2017).

[1] From another perspective, 43.4% of people who are involved in the sexual activities on-screen and online are found to be married, though the main motivation for this may not solely be lust or addiction, but more so as a profession and monetary gain (Brown et al., 2017).

Introduction:

"Samir doesn't know how to express his love for me, or so I believed. Nearly three years into our marriage, it is always me who initiates romantic gestures, if you know what I mean." Samia, Samir's wife disclosed this to me during one of our counselling sessions. She has observed Samir's seclusion, sleepless nights, and coldness when it comes to verbal or physical romantic expressions. "It was disheartening to see him be vibrant with his friends and other family members, but frigid and emotionally distant with me," Samia contines. "Until one night, when I was in excruciating stomach pain in the middle of the night, I literally shrieked in agony. I believed Samir was sleeping, so I called out to him to wake up and help me, but he was not in bed. I literally crawled out of bed, like a soldier

135

on the battlefield, until I exited my bedroom, then I heard Samir's voice emanating from another room, and dragged my body towards his voice—but then I was shaken to the core."

Samir was having an online conversation with an escort worker with his pants down. "Not only was he experiencing sexual fantasies and gratification, but he was also expressing his interests, emotions, and awe at the beauty of the woman he was talking with. My pain came to a sudden standstill," Samia said while gazing at the walls with her eyes wide open and tears streaming down her face. "It felt as if my entire existence had come to a complete stop, to the point where I was unable to even call him for help or make him feel that I had caught him in his shame."

Samia also narrated that his computer screen was divided into two pages, one where he was talking to the sex worker while enjoying her dirty lead, and the other containing pornographic images that they were both sharing to spice up their filthy activity.

As Samia continued to tell her story, I realized that his coldness towards her was a result of his involvement in porn consumption and his desire to find sexual pleasure elsewhere. It is unsurprising that he had no interest in romantic or sexual intimacy with his wife.

Etiology

Relationship status has been a vital factor in the porn-seeking behavior of people. Whether they are coping with an ongoing bad relationship or looking for a specific factor that they cannot satisfy with their current partner, porn addicts find ways to justify their actions, despite being in a stable relationship already. Whatever the reason, emotional detachment is almost always the expected outcome.

1. **Growing apart.** In some cohorts, couples grow colder through time and therefore have much lesser physical contact and sexual activity, which can result in porn-seeking behavior (Brown et al., 2017). In fact, a previous statistic has shown that the leading cause of divorce among married partners include growing apart (55%) and not being able to talk to their partner (53%), which are all possible manifestations of emotional detachment (Scott et al, 2013). If partnered individuals once have enjoyed the warmth of a good relationship, they are bound to seek a consistent feeling of love and care. But in porn addicts, satisfaction is more than love and care. With the hunger of a porn addict for gratification, the warmth of a loving relationship may not be sufficient, and thus can cause them to grow apart from their partners.

2. **One-sided relationships.** Another person significantly affected by emotional detachment from a porn addict, is their partner themselves. According to a study, marital partners who are dependent on pornography use may feel one-sidedness in their relationship, losing the sense of effort from their porn-addicted partners and therefore lose interest themselves (De Alarcón et al., 2019). A porn addict may lose focus on their responsibilities as a part of a relationship, which transfers heavier responsibilities to their partner. While their partners may be patient, tolerating this behavior may result in long-term and irreparable problems.

3. **Domestic violence.** Emotional detachment is not always the dead silence of indifference between partners, but also may manifest as a violent behavior from the partner. From

various studies, porn addiction can possibly lead to mood swings, aggressive behavior, and even hostility towards their partners. In research on once-committed individuals, 23.5% of the divorced people from the study confessed that domestic violence is an important etiology of separation in married people (Scott, et al., 2013). Though there are limited studies on porn addiction and domestic violence, this is a possible trajectory of being invested in sexually explicit materials that tolerate demeaning and harming partners for sex.

4. **Disagreements.** Conflicts are thought to be a normal part of a relationship. However, arguments are difficult to mediate when one partner has a conflict with their neuropsychological, cognitive, and socio-personal standpoint. Porn addicts may not be the best parties engaged in an argument due to the broad symptomatology brought about by their addiction, ranging from the conflict with their social skills, uncertainty in their psychological presentations, and decreased cognitive function. When arguments in relationships become worse, they are bound to result in emotional detachment. In a study, arguments and conflicts in relationships are found to be important reasons for divorce (Scott et al., 2013). If applied to the porn addict, their predisposition to unorthodox ways, more so as a part of a relationship, can put themselves at risk for these disagreements and eventually emotional detachment.

Relationships involving a porn addict usually would include a combination of moral dilemmas, social constraints, potential loss of trust, and a high risk of emotional detachment.

Epidemiology

Pornography addiction and its effects on committed relationships is a broad topic that does not have that much focus and exposure yet. Nevertheless, it has been thought that continuous use of online pornography may result in emotional detachment trouble which can affect your overall capacity to build healthier relationships (De Alarcón et al., 2019).

Around 22-76% of manifestations of hypersexuality include having multiple romantic relationships, including other hypersexual behavior such as compulsive cruising, promiscuity, and lack of control in using pornography (De Alarcón et al., 2019). Once these individuals who engage in chronic porn usage become part of a committed relationship, they may have inherent hypersexuality brought about by the nature of their addiction. These can lead to the said behavior, which can ultimately lead to emotional detachment.

Once successful, porn addicts may not have a smooth course of a relationship, while still engaging in long-term porn use. Their actions may grow latent feelings of shame, which may have collateral damage to their partners. In a study, people, who identify as scrupulous and disapproved of porn use, have felt great shame in using porn and were found to have the tendency to blame their habits on others (Volk et al., 2019). Upon admission of addiction, they have the tendency to blame their partners, in most cases, their wives, finding ways to look for any faults in others that might've caused their addiction, which worsens their emotional detachment in the long run.

In some cases of pornography use, addiction starts out late in their lives, when they are already married. In once-married individuals, divorced people are found to have a 25% higher chance of seeking pornographic material than single people (Brown et al., 2017). One of their motivations is to substitute the affection that they do not receive any more and may have longed for after being in a committed relationship.

We must note here that confounding factors may make future studies difficult as the performance of a porn addict as a romantic partner is not solely dependent on their current factors. It should be noted that most of these porn addicts have a psychologically significant history that can make it difficult for them to work in a committed relationship, despite finding their preferred partner.

Severing emotional attachments: How porn addiction ruins relationships

As commonly studied, addiction takes its toll on the brain first, where prolonged addiction results in dysfunction of the normal neurophysiology of the brain, which results in a restructuring of the overall brain anatomy (Flores, 2006). These biological mechanisms will naturally result in psychosocial implications, which if manifested while in a committed relationship, may result in emotional detachment from their partners.

While the exact pathophysiology of porn addiction has not been explained from an individual to a relationship standpoint, few studies have ventured into the points of view of individuals who are in a relationship with porn addicts. One study has found three attachment-related influences of online pornography use and deception by husbands as felt by their respective wives (Zitzman & Butler, 2009).

1. The initial growth of an attachment fault line in their commitment, which roots in the perceived attachment infidelity. At a certain moment within the timeline of addiction, porn use not only serves as the root source of the fault line but also serves as a coping mechanism to possibly cover their own interpersonal faults (Flores, 2006). The long-term problem of porn use cannot be easily removed from one's habits in order to adjust to their partners' needs, and therefore may call for more drastic management (Zitzman, & Butler, 2009). Meanwhile, not all people treat porn addiction as a condition, and thus treat it as a form of attachment infidelity, which dents their relationship.

2. The development of the gap in the attachment rift arises from a partner's feeling of distance from their respective partner. For porn addicts, the relationship would be difficult to manage as well, which results in their loss of confidence in their partner and their relationship, as well as the continuous deterioration of the brain from these activities (Zitzman, & Butler, 2009). The forming distance and disconnection from the porn-addicted partners are expected to grow further if not managed early.

3. Formation of attachment estrangement secondary to the worsening lack of emotional and psychological security from their partner. While in a normal relationship, people find a sense of comfort and security from their partner, people who have porn addicts as partners may eventually lose their proper emotional regulatory function while with them (Zitzman, & Butler, 2009). While this can be resolved by itself through trust and communication, solving the porn addiction must be the paramount concern as this may result in recurrence or relapse, psychological co-morbidities for both partners, and worse relationship outcomes.

This evolution of the pathology of emotional detachment is one of the primary reasons why porn addicts are in unstable relationships. The affected people are less likely to effectively maintain a healthy bond with another person during the course of their addiction. If they happen to be in one, the relationship may tend to be exploitative, maladaptive, and sadomasochistic (Flores, 2006). From young people committed in a relationship up to married individuals, porn addiction may result in long-term complications for both members of the party, if not resolved early.

Psychosocial manifestations of emotional detachment

Unlike other conditions, emotional detachment in people who engaged in long-term pornography use is difficult to quantify due to the overlap in other related conditions, such as hypersexual behavior.

Sexual dissatisfaction. Sexual dissatisfaction in partnered individuals is one of the manifestations found to be instrumental in the emotional detachment of people involving porn addicts. Sexual dissatisfaction can be observed both in the porn addict and their partner. Relationships can tend to be one-sided, where only one person benefits the most, more than the other (De Alarcón, et al., 2019). This can translate to the quality of their sexual relationship, which may also turn out one-sided. This is bound to problems in the relationship, having internal sentiments that may not initially reveal their dissatisfaction with their status. This may be the root of a growing problem, especially if they see themselves as long-term partners. Decreased quality of relationship and sexual satisfaction, according to a study, is parallel to relationship dissatisfaction with a partner engaged in substance abuse (Pyle, & Bridges, 2012).

Promiscuity. Commitment in a monogamous relationship may not be completely ideal for the porn addict as they have the tendency to be promiscuous (De Alarcón, et al., 2019). The hypersexual behavior of porn addicts is a huge part of their personality as chronic porn consumers, which entails sexually adventurous and potentially sexually inappropriate activities. Promiscuity, even in a person who is committed to a partner, may not be an indication of an ideal mate. This urge to engage in sexual activity, sometimes with people unknown to them or to their partners, may be difficult to control, despite the confines of romantic commitment. As this is a part of hypersexual behavior, the management of this may aim for the salvage of their relationship.

Infidelity secondary to multiple relationships. It is a significant part of the pathology of the porn addict, where they continue to seek more sources of gratification and can develop tolerance to one sex object (De Alarcón, et al., 2019). Therefore, a porn addict, who is in a relationship, may develop urges to seek more options to date and experiment with. These will eventually lead to sexual infidelity. While at first, this may seem like an adventure for them, this actually feeds their addiction further, because porn has already remodeled their brain to seek pleasure, even in the most unorthodox manner. Much worse is when the porn addict gets themselves into multiple relationships, which broadens the number of emotionally damaging consequences towards more people.

Higher secrecy of porn use. Secrecy of porn use from one's partner was found to be one of the most significant factors in relationship dissatisfaction, along with the frequency of use of pornography (Pyle & Bridges, 2012). Using pornography while in a relationship may be suggestive of something lacking in the relationship and has shown negative reactions from their partners. While committed relationships are a good avenue for consensual sex, porn addicts do not seek the safety of sexual relationships, but rather the dopamine boost that they need to get them through the day. Porn habits by an addict are most likely under the covers and are unknown to the partner, despite having a strong bond. This does not completely entail a loss of trust on behalf of the porn addict, as this may be a manifestation of the shame felt from consuming porn by the addict. However, this may not be completely understood by their romantic partners, no matter how patient they are with their loved ones.

While more manifestations of a porn addiction may be reflective of emotional detachment, they still need further studies to objectively assess these symptoms. The challenge in assessing emotional detachment is that it may overlap with other conditions, such as clinical depression, anxiety disorders, and even personality disorders.

Porn use as an adaptation on emotional detachment

When porn serves as a coping mechanism, the porn addict can justify their behavior in a myriad of ways that can make them feel secured with tolerating porn consumption. This can be expected in people who use porn as an adaptation to a loss of warmth from a previous relationship or an interrupted one. In fact, in one study of 357 adults, the use of pornography is indeed rationalized to be a coping mechanism for the deprivation of human affection (Hesse & Floyd, 2019).

The efficacy of porn as an adaptation to emotional detachment is straightforward. The brain is usually looking for a source of pleasure, satisfaction, and even affection, one that is now deprived of them after emotional detachment. Because porn offers a quick boost of dopamine, it has become a famous avenue for people who would like to cope with their own problems. In a study, pornography use has been associated with substitution for the affection they once had from their partner (Hesse & Floyd, 2019).

Because emotional detachment calls for a resolution with their partners and even the formation of a new one with another individual, solving their problems on their own is not an easy feat to do. With just several clicks from their computer mouse, the World Wide Web opens some more options to observe and potentially manifest with a non-existential emotional warmth. As the porn industry displays its actors as charismatic, they may be the perfect image for someone who can provide their sexual needs unconditionally, without the effort needed to maintain an actual human relationship.

Repairing emotional detachment in porn addicts

Because of the nature of the activity, pornographic consumption is a difficult part of a lifestyle to accept and resolve, even with a committed romantic partner. Because of the distrust that it makes a partner feel as well as the secrecy of the habit itself, porn addicts who are in a committed relationship are likely to be tackling these problems by themselves. However, pornographic addiction alone is a difficult condition to resolve, more so if there is another person at risk of being affected by the outcome. Nevertheless, carefully structured resolution plans are the ideal management, in cooperation with their respective partners.

The primary goal of the management is to repair the healthy relationship if the partner agrees to undergo the management with the affected person. Specific goals of the management include earning the trust of the partner, assuring adequacy in affection amongst partners, and the overall resolution of pornography addiction.

Primarily, the porn addict must be made aware of their detrimental habit, which can affect them and their respective partners. If the partner is still in the picture, they should ideally be a part of the management, for them to see and appreciate the effort on how to recover from this condition. This potentially re-establishes sympathy from one partner to the other, as well as sparking camaraderie between them. In a study, people who are involved in heavy pornographic use while being in a romantic relationship were found to have treatment-seeking behavior, in an effort to recover from porn addiction and be better partners (Bergner & Bridges, 2002). Partners of porn addicts must be informed of this as well, to let them know that treatment-seeking behavior is a good indication of treatment success.

Regaining the trust of people who are closest to the porn addict is vital in repairing once-healthy relationships (De Alarcón et al., 2019). Trust is vital for improving the odds of success. The best way to establish this is for the porn addict to finally step up and be proactive in controlling their porn consumption urges. To emphasize the importance of stopping chronic porn use, it must be noted that psychology researchers acknowledged that addiction is inversely correlated with the capacity to form healthy relationships (Flores, 2006). Therefore, an effort to carefully stop the habit of porn consumption must be initiated as early as possible. Gradual withdrawal from the addiction may be much more bearable than in people who do not have anyone to support them, like married individuals, young adults who are exclusively dating, or even those in a strictly committed relationship. In fact, it was noted that people have been found to consume 20 percent less pornography once they are legally committed (Brown et al., 2017). Once successful, this can improve their chances of regaining their partner's trust, while being able to manage the root of their problem, which is the porn addiction itself.

Addiction has been known to induce a rush of satisfying emotions that numbs the individual of the more subtle emotions in life. Consequently, these affected individuals let these valuable emotional feelings be a substitute for addiction (Flores, 2006). In order to prevent relapse from these, both the recovering addict and their respective partner must assure open communication with regard to their emotions, in order to inform their partner of their problems, and what they need at the moment. Overall, this can increase the chances of repairing the relationship, from the aspects of trust, communication, and affection, once and for all.

References:
[1] Brown, C. C., Durtschi, J. A., Carroll, J. S., & Willoughby, B. J. (2017). *Understanding and predicting classes of college students who use pornography.* Computers in Human Behavior, 66, 114–121.
[2] Butler, M. H., Pereyra, S. A., Draper, T. W., Leonhardt, N. D., & Skinner, K. B. (2018). *Pornography use and loneliness: A bidirectional recursive model and pilot investigation.* Journal of Sex and Marital Therapy, 44(2), 127–137. doi:10.1080/0092623X.2017.1321601
[3] Yoder, V. C., Virden, T. B., & Amin, K. (2005). *Internet pornography and loneliness: An association?.* Sexual Addiction & Compulsivity, 12, 19–44. doi:10.1080/10720160590933653
Volk, F., Floyd, C. G., Bohannon, K. E., Cole, S. M., McNichol, K. M., Schott, E. A., & Williams, Z. D. R. (2019). *The Moderating Role of the Tendency to Blame Others in the Development of Perceived Addiction, Shame, and Depression in Pornography Users.* Sexual Addiction & Compulsivity, 1–23. doi:10.1080/10720162.2019.1670301
De Alarcón, R., de la Iglesia, J., Casado, N., & Montejo, A. (2019). *Online Porn Addiction: What We Know and What We Don't—A Systematic Review.* Journal of Clinical Medicine, 8(1), 91. doi:10.3390/jcm8010091
Pyle, T. M., & Bridges, A. J. (2012). *Perceptions of relationship satisfaction and addictive behavior: Comparing pornography and marijuana use.* Journal of Behavioral Addictions, 1(4), 171–179. doi:10.1556/jba.1.2012.007

Zitzman, S. T., & Butler, M. H. (2009). *Wives' Experience of Husbands' Pornography Use and Concomitant Deception as an Attachment Threat in the Adult Pair-Bond Relationship.* Sexual Addiction & Compulsivity, 16(3), 210–240. doi:10.1080/10720160903202679

Flores, P. J. (2006). *Conflict and Repair in Addiction Treatment. Journal of Groups in Addiction & Recovery, 1(1), 5–26.* doi:10.1300/j384v01n01_02

Scott, S. B., Rhoades, G. K., Stanley, S. M., Allen, E. S., & Markman, H. J. (2013). *Reasons for divorce and recollections of premarital intervention: Implications for improving relationship education. Couple and Family Psychology: Research and Practice, 2(2), 131–145.* doi:10.1037/a0032025

Hesse, C., & Floyd, K. (2019). *Affection substitution: The effect of pornography consumption on close relationships. Journal of Social and Personal Relationships, 026540751984171.* doi:10.1177/0265407519841719

Bergner, R. M., & Bridges, A. J. (2002). *The Significance of Heavy Pornography Involvement for Romantic Partners: Research and Clinical Implications. Journal of Sex & Marital Therapy, 28(3), 193–206.* doi:10.1080/009262302760328235

Ch.11

Porn & decision impairment

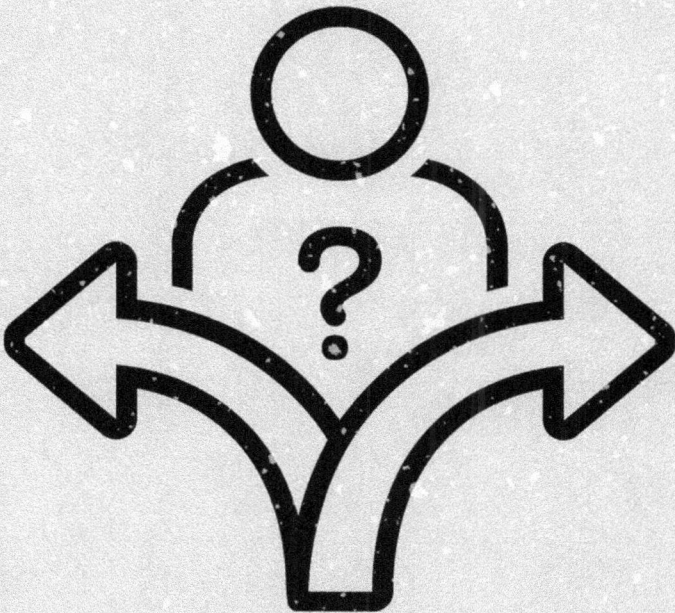

How can pornography lead to the inability to make sound decisions?

Introduction:

Jeremy, a 45-year-old former CEO of his own company, had sought a consultation with a psychiatrist to clear up an embarrassing issue for him, bothering him since he was a young child. This problem has cost him his loving wife, successful business, and even his valued peace of mind. Now while being aware of his problem, he is still as helpless as ever.

When he was 7 years old, Jeremy had seen his father having sex with his mistress. The graphic image of them in different contorting positions while breathing fast and hard had always bothered him as a child. It was not arousing or disgusting to him at that time. It was merely confusing. It was something that he thinks feels good but is also wrong. He did not know what had happened, but he knew that it was something that he cannot talk to anyone about. From then on, it remained a confusing memory.

Lacking comprehension at that time, he was never exposed to anything sexual or romantic in nature as his parents are not expressive of their love if there are still feelings. As an only child, he never had siblings to ask about these feelings that confused him. After all, four years later, his parents got divorced, which widened the gap between his mom and dad even further. In the mind of a young boy, these mature matters are not something that can be processed well yet.

After school, he spent most of his time at home, surfing the internet, playing games, and streaming online videos. On the website he was playing at, he saw an extremely graphic advertisement showing a short, looped video of a naked woman with heaving bosoms, seductively winking at him. This had sparked a new and curious coping mechanism, one that he thought he needed since he was a needy child. The day had become a core memory to him, as that was when he saw a video showing an older man in a suit and tie, being seduced by his secretary, which had clarified his memory of his father with another woman. This started an entire rabbit hole of pornographic content that he kept scrolling and consuming. As he watches intently, he never bothered to look at the clock. This had become an after-school habit of his, watching pornography all day. From then on, he had skipped a lot of football practices at school, enough to get him kicked out of the team. He also had much lower grades at school. He never really cared about these or anything else in the world, as long as he is seated in his swivel chair, with one hand on his mouse, and another on his young body. This had continued until his adulthood, being married to a wonderful woman his father had chosen for him, for the purpose of expansion of their respective family businesses. Jeremy also took over his dad's position as the CEO of their family company. Despite all of the inherited success, he had a carefree life outside his home and a private life inside his room.

One early morning, he was in the master bathroom, pleasuring himself while his eyes are glued to his smart phone screen. He naturally turns off any notifications, calls, or messages, so that nothing can interrupt his morning ritual in the bathroom. It turned out that he was receiving almost hundreds of missed calls from his colleagues and employees at work. It turned out that they had lost a great number of valuable spools of golden wires in the manufacturing department, and they need Jeremy's authorization to inspect the office, as they suspect the thief was still there. Jeremy arrived at work before lunch, and headed to the cafeteria to eat, before proceeding to his office. He started his workday at 1:00 pm, missing almost half a day of his business's operational hours. And most of all, he had missed the fiasco early that morning, where his authority was needed to make executive decisions for the encountered problem. Upon inspection, the thief was caught on camera packing the golden wires, leaving the premises before lunch as he claimed that he is from the night shift, going home. Jeremy recognized the thief's face, as he was supposed to be with him during regular random inspections, to prevent these incidences of looting. The news spread like wildfire. While not the primary suspect for the problem, Jeremy had gained an irresponsible reputation, going to work late, and leaving it early as well. While he could have prevented the scenarios, he remained adherent to his habits of pornographic use. This had prompted Jeremy's father-in-law to have to divorce his wife, because of the many mistakes that had unraveled due to the problem. Upon learning of Jeremy's porn addiction, his wife did not take it well and decided to leave him. This had encouraged him to seek treatment already, to see the problem, and hopefully find a permanent solution.

Etiology of decision impairment in porn addicts

Decision impairment is apparent in people afflicted with addiction. While the potential factors contributing to these are known, including neurological, psychological, and socio-personal factors, the outcomes of decision-making are not yet well-studied in porn addicts.

Poor executive planning and function. The executive functioning of the brain is what separates humans from other organisms. This function is expected to develop rapidly since childhood. However, when a neuropsychological phenomenon interrupts this function, it may derail the intellectual development of the person. Pornographic addiction, along with other forms of behavioral and substance addiction, has been found to be related to a gradual decline in cognition. In the field of behavioral research, the **Interaction of Person-Affect-Cognition-Execution (I-PACE) theoretical framework** is used in various studies to assess people afflicted by addiction, including problematic pornographic use, and cognition and execution as factors (Brand et al., 2019). This study model strongly considers decision impairment as a possible factor that strengthens the risk of pornographic addiction. An overall decline in cognitive function results in a weaker foundation to make good decisions in life.

Change in behaviors brought about by chronic porn use. The avenue for continuous use of anything addictive, besides the executive function and effortful control, is compulsive and impulsive behavior. A study has presented the **Cyber pornography addiction test (CYPAT)**, as well as other pre-existing psychometric tests for porn addicts, which takes into account the compulsive behavior of the subjects (Cacioppo et al., 2018). Compulsive sexual behavior leads to engagement in spontaneous activities for sexual gratification, without considering the risks accompanying it. Compulsion contributes to the lack of control in craving for sexual satisfaction, which leads to chronic pornographic use. As described by Bensimon (2007), pornographic addiction is fueled by compulsive behavior in two steps: 1) **compulsive dependence** on pornographic use, and 2) the **repeated failure** to recover from the condition, upon awareness of it. While some pornographic users acknowledge this compulsive behavior and its respective consequences, it does not guarantee treatment-seeking behavior.

Shifting priorities to make way for regular porn use. Porn addiction, similar to other forms of addiction, predisposes the individual to seek the immediate pleasures of porn and sex. People afflicted with addiction manifest with excessive delay discounting, which is when a person consistently discounts the value of the delayed rewards, to prioritize instant but temporary pleasures (Koffarnus & Kaplan, 2018). This emphasizes the natural tendency of porn addicts to shift their priorities to achieve near-term rewards, such as the high one gets from using drugs, as compared to long-term rewards, such as stable interpersonal relationships (Koffarnus & Kaplan, 2018). In the long run, their pleasure-seeking ways will compromise their personal goals and will compromise their overall satisfaction in life.

The pathological need for sexual gratification from porn. People who have a substance addiction value drug-related rewards, more than other forms of reward (Koffarnus & Kaplan, 2018). This is parallel to the manifestations of behavioral addicts, such as those with pornographic addiction. This reflects how they prioritize the goal of sustaining sexual craving (i.e., satisfaction secondary to pornographic use), over what is needed for a better life (e.g., studying, exercising, etc.). This will then affect their decision-making and daily planning, in order to make way for their pornographic use, despite their busy schedule. Not only does it take precious time away from these individuals, but pornographic use will also ruin their motivational centers to do things that matter.

This may come as a challenge to the researchers of today as they have to deal with a number of confounding factors that contribute to poor decision-making skills, such as intelligence quotient, life experiences, and even being street-smart. In spite of this, a study was conducted to find out how to objectively assess decision-making skills in people who are engaged in substance and behavioral addiction (Koffarnus & Kaplan, 2018). From managing reward systems to changes in personality, many mechanisms contribute to how pornography addicts end up becoming bad decision-makers.

Pathophysiology: The psychology of bad decisions in porn addicts

Establishment of chronic porn consumption guarantees the continuous exposure of the brain and body to the unearned set of rewards from the dose of dopamine boost up to the temporal pleasure people get from the experience. Its effect on decision-making skills, however, includes a more complex umbrella of mechanisms, from a decline in motivation, various changes in priorities, and the dreaded long-term consequences of bad decisions.

The habit loop serves as a simple yet effective presentation of how the habit of pornographic consumption takes place. The depicted sexual stimulus, brought about by digital pornographic materials, serves as a starting point for a habit. These arousing stimuli denote action, which is through watching porn and gratifying oneself with it, which embodies a pleasurable experience for the individual. Because of the effect of pornographic use on the person, they have expected the reward of a dopamine boost, which prompts them to do it all over again. Cognitive functions do not function well when the pleasure centers of the brain are already in-charge of the priorities. With this in mind, these people still commit to consuming porn, regardless of its long-term consequences. This results in an almost endless cycle of stimulation, pornographic consumption, and dopamine reward. Eventually, this will initiate a pleasure-seeking habit that is now the start of an addiction. However, this is not sustainable.

Pornography consumption is a time-consuming hobby. Taking time to use pornography is the first of the many bad decision these people commit to, and it paves the road to chronic porn use. It takes up precious time to accommodate all of the activities that it entails: from initiating and maintaining arousal, one's energy focuses on initiating a response that is supposed to be partially involuntary. Searching for pornographic content is similar to the endless rabbit hole of searching through social media, where one can go scrolling for hours without noticing how much time they are already taking. In other people, another challenge is the numerous pornographic content to choose from, which can take too much time to explore all while potentially inducing decision fatigue in the user. This can go on for hours, without the person looking at the time. This seemingly unlimited time allotted for pornography use is common, to the point that they can miss other scheduled activities and be late on their commitments. With higher frequency, this can manifest as constant tardiness, which prompts the person to create excuses to justify their punctuality issues and maintain their porn consumption activities. This can develop into a habit and can be a part of their lifestyle already, which finally establishes the addiction.

These psychosocial manifestations are not limited to habits and lifestyle – they also affect the neurobiological structures and functions. Multiple studies have looked into the brains of chronic porn users, finding several structures to have lesser gray matter volume and weaker brain connections between various structures (De Sousa & Lodha, 2017). These neuroanatomical changes result in changes in the production and regulation of serotonin, and the resulting serotonin/dopamine ratio, which can manifest as behavioral changes. Some of these include behaviors of sexual nature, e.g., erotic excitability, hypersexuality, and predisposition to online porn addiction, as well as cognitive manifestations, e.g., depression, interpersonal sensitivity, and a longer time needed to recover from the addiction. Among the most pertinent reported symptoms from the hypersexual subjects of the study is the overall deteriorated executive function (De Sousa & Lodha, 2017). In addition to this, working memory is gravely impaired as a result of sexual arousal induced by viewing digital pornographic content. Switching and monitoring performance is affected as well, which is considered to contribute to the deficits in maintaining attention. All of these contribute significantly to the overall decline in the executive function of porn addicts, which debilitates their capacity to make good decisions.

Clinical manifestations: How do porn addicts create bad decisions

Dysfunction in decision-making is a straightforward manifestation, as compared to other portions of the pathology of pornography addiction. Despite this, there are several considerations in assessing problems in decision-making. This is important to further qualify if the manifestation is indeed secondary to porn addiction, or to another etiology.

Disarrayed executive function and planning. Porn addicts always make way for sexual gratification in their daily priorities, thus allotting time for an intensive porn consumption and self-gratification, while leaving much less time for things they actually need to do. They give much less attention to real-life matters, thus taking a toll on their efficiency in occupation and personal life. They end up losing touch with their responsibilities. Furthermore, this aggravates the deteriorating quality of their decisions. Because the executive function is vital to the formation of the most rational plan for a specific situation, the mind of a porn addict is not the best fit for planning complex matters. The problem with this is that, because of the neuroanatomical and physiological changes in the brain, the proper cognition of the porn addict is not expected to be back in a healthy shape even after a good night's rest (De Sousa & Lodha, 2017). The neurobiological state of the individual is expected to take a long time to improve and the person would have to proactively change their ways, recover from pornographic addiction, and wait for the rewiring of the brain to take place, while living with the current consequences of poorer executive function.

Lower effortful control. Research confirmed that executive function is poorer in subjects who are engaged in problematic pornography use, especially involving their general control of their behavior, inhibitions, and motivations (Okabe, Takahashi & Ito, 2021). The components of executive function were carefully assessed and showed congruent results. Among these is the lower effortful control in the subjects who have problematic pornography use, meaning their capacity to have attention control, inhibitory control, and activation control, as measured using the Effortful Control (EC) scale of the Adult Temperament Questionnaire (Rothbart, Ahadi & Evans, 2000). Attention control pertains to the capacity of the person to focus on a specific task, especially when in distress. Unfortunately, in porn addicts, attention is compromised thus manifesting as a poor focus on things that matter. Inhibitory control is comprised of the intrinsic self-discipline to fight cravings. Being under any form of addiction is a giveaway that the particular person has failed in this aspect. And lastly, activation control consists of the capacity of the person to proactively initiate a task despite not having adequate motivation for it. While most people wait for their motivation to kick in before partaking in a task, the porn addict does not have any motivation to accomplish anything, regardless of the level of urgency. Overall, the study correlated the lack of effortful control to the compulsive behavior of these people, which puts them at risk for addiction and difficulty in recovery (Rothbart, Ahadi & Evans, 2000).

Excessive delay discounting. As part of a good approach to decision-making, weighing the pros and cons of a decision should be done to assure the best outcomes for any situation. Because of their compromised executive function, porn addicts may not be the best people to plan a great strategy. Because time is of the essence in most, if not all, situations, predicting good outcomes for delayed actions as compared to doing actions at present is a necessary approach to decision-making. In lieu of this, delay discounting is a tell-tale sign of bad behavior, which can branch out to other faults in socio-personal manifestations. Also known as temporal discounting, this behavior engrains much less value on a future goal than on one at present, which contributes to poor decision-making in people at risk of addiction (Duan, Wu & Sun, 2017). The problem with this is that their compulsion also prevents them from having the discipline to wait for a particular moment to get better outcomes than getting a reward here and now. As a component of impulsivity, delay discounting in normal people is a good predictor of a tendency to engage in addicting behavior and difficulty in recovering once they are already in the rabbit hole of cyclic engagement in porn use (Koffarnus & Kaplan, 2018).

Management

Decision impairment entails much longer management, due to the nature of its pathology, involving neurobiological changes that may need time to happen. The immediate goal of management is to resolve the pornography addiction once and for all, to repair pre-existing problems in their lives, and to prevent falling back into the same patterns as before.

Quitting pornography is a very difficult feat, as it usually has been interwoven with their daily lifestyle. However, this is one of the most vital parts of the treatment goals, because this cuts the root of all the evils of an addict. Withdrawal can be painful as one must push their body to the limit, in order to prevent them from engaging in unearned dopamine and serotonin-boosting activities. This can be done gradually to prevent relapse.

While these are happening, make sure that the affected person knows basic social skills, so that they can repair whatever relationship or matter that are still reparable. Fixing broken friendships is also not easy, but communication is key to having a better friend. This emphasizes that some relationships that have broken up due to pornography addiction, may have the possibility of renewal. Also, this reminds the affected person that they may need other people to recover from such events.

All of these can strengthen the condition of the person affected. With prolonged abstinence from pornography, these people can have brain changes brought about by withdrawal from pornographic consumption, which is one of the first effects that can be observed in real-life.

References:
Koffarnus, M. N., & Kaplan, B. A. (2018). *Clinical models of decision making in addiction. Pharmacology Biochemistry and Behavior, 164,* 71–83. *doi:10.1016/j.pbb.2017.08.010*
Duan, J., Wu, S. J., & Sun, L. (2017). *Do the Powerful Discount the Future Less? The Effects of Power on Temporal Discounting. Frontiers in Psychology, 8. doi:10.3389/fpsyg.2017.01007*
Brand, M., Wegmann, E., Stark, R., Müller, A., Wölfling, K., Robbins, T. W., & Potenza, M. N. (2019). *The Interaction of Person-Affect-Cognition-Execution (I-PACE) model for addictive behaviors: Update, generalization to addictive behaviors beyond Internet-use disorders, and specification of the process character of addictive behaviors. Neuroscience & Biobehavioral Reviews. doi:10.1016/j.neubiorev.2019.06.032*

Okabe Y, Takahashi F, & Ito D. (2021). Problematic Pornography Use in Japan: A Preliminary Study Among University Students. Front Psychol. Apr 16;12:638354. doi: 10.3389/fpsyg.2021.638354. PMID: 33935889; PMCID: PMC8085335.

Rothbart M. K., Ahadi S. A., Evans D. E. (2000). Temperament and personality: origins and outcomes. J. Personal Soc. Psychol. 78 122–135. 10.1037/0022-3514.78.1.122

Cacioppo, M., Gori, A., Schimmenti, A., Baiocco, R., Laghi, F., & Caretti, V. (2018). Development of a new screening tool for cyber pornography: Psychometric properties of the Cyber Pornography Addiction Test (CYPAT). Clinical neuropsychiatry, 15(1).

Bensimon, P. (2007). The Role of Pornography in Sexual Offending. Sexual Addiction & Compulsivity, 14(2), 95–117. doi:10.1080/10720160701310468

De Sousa, A., & Lodha, P. (2017). Neurobiology of Pornography Addiction–A clinical review. Telangana journal of psychiatry, 3(2), 66.

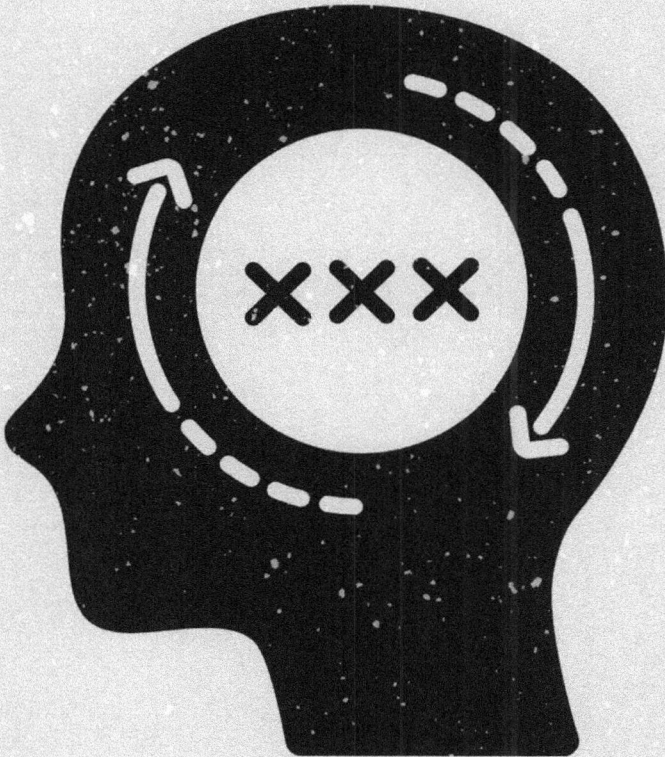

Ch.12

Porn & addiction

Addiction is a brain disease

Key points discussed in this chapter:

[1] According to some people who are regular consumers of pornographic materials, their primary motivation includes the development of their real-life sexual interaction, probably through visualization of possible sexual activities they can undertake.

[1] Another motivation includes substitution for their non-existential sexual relationship, which allows them to feel sexual sensations that they cannot feel in a real-life relationship with a consensual partner.

[2] Technically, pornography addiction is a part of a larger group of mental disorders involved in sexual addiction. Nevertheless, having one condition involving sexual addiction is likely to be correlated to the development of pornography addiction.

[2] As frequent consumption of porn materials can result in problems with self-control and can disrupt normal daily life, it is regarded as a brain pathological problem that requires medical intervention. The involvement of neurotransmitters and their disequilibrium affects the normal functions of the human and can result in abnormal responses to stimuli, such as hypersensitivity to sexual and non-sexual cues, fatigue, and grave loss of concentration.

[3] Pornographic addiction is classified under impulse control behavior through the International Classification of Diseases 11th Revision (ICD-11). However, further studies should be done to analyze the sexual component of pornographic addiction as this may entail different levels of disruptions in neurotransmitters and may affect behavior differently.

[3] Pornographic addiction can potentially result in maladaptive behaviors that put the person at risk for more health and life-threatening risks.

Introduction

The paradigm shift in the psychological aspect of addiction has opened the acceptance of behavioral addiction. Studies on substance addiction paved the way for how people are predisposed to cravings, compulsions, tolerance, dependence, and long-term chronic use. Despite this, porn addiction is still not a diagnosable illness.

In *The Diagnostic and Statistical Manual of Mental Disorders* by the American Psychiatric Association (2022), it is only classified under the Hypersexuality Disorder, while the International Classification of Diseases by the World Health Organization (2019) identified similar behavior as compulsive sexual behavior. Unlike voyeurism or exhibitionism, the consumption of pornographic material still does not belong under sexual conditions (American Psychiatric Association, 2022). Despite the increasing number of studies and cases reported, as of today, pornographic addiction as a single disease entity is not yet published in the authority when it comes to diseases.

Considering this, addiction to porn consumption needs to be recognized as a separate condition. Pornographic addiction encompasses a combination of hypersexuality, unregulated internet usage, and an overall lack of self-control. In fact, a study compared the degree of effect of pornographic addiction to marijuana use in a romantic relationship, which showed significant similarities between substance abuse to behavioral addiction (Pyle & Bridges, 2012). This can reflect on the similarity in the pathophysiology of behavioral and substance addiction, with the main difference just being their stimuli while they activate the same reward via the pleasure pathway.

The objectives of this chapter is to discuss the pertinent details of pornographic addiction such as the etiology and epidemiology, elaborate the biopsychological implications of the condition, e.g., pathophysiology and clinical manifestation, and advise an effective management plan to control, reduce, and stop pornography use once and for all.

Etiology

Behavioral addiction usually comes from a relevant painful history, further aggravated by socio-personal, family, and environmental factors. With the sensitive nature of pornographic addiction, an affliction related to sexual trauma is also expected. The etiology and risk factors of pornographic addiction can be correlated with a need to satisfy oneself sexually, without the benefit of a consenting romantic sexual partner. The need for this usually comes naturally through age, from the curiosity of the adolescent to the inherent need for physical stimulation of the adult in their reproductive age. While having sexual needs is normal, an intense need for sexual gratification can reach pathological degrees. Because not all people have the benefit of easily getting into a romantic relationship to find a sexual partner, some people may have to resort to more unconventional measures of sexual gratification without having the need to find a partner. The following are some of the possible causes and risk factors for people to get caught in the trap of pornographic addiction.

History of psychological pain. Most people have their own psychological struggles, most especially during childhood. Granted that we all have our own challenges in life, not all people are well-equipped to handle these problems. Some of these people are unfortunate to come from broken families, or those with unhealthy familial attachments. Some of these people are on the receiving end of intense forms of emotional abuse such as gaslighting, manipulation, or breadcrumbing. Some people may be trapped in an emotionally abusive relationship with their parents, siblings, or even extended family members. In adults, they may be locked in a frustrating relationship.

Some people are led to some easily accessible forms of satisfaction, without the need to take the effort of normal social convention. For people with significant psychological struggles, pornographic addiction can serve as an anesthetic to mentally unbearable pain. In addition to this, they also gain pleasure from it, feeling good about themselves despite everything that is happening to them (Coleman, 1987). While pleasure hormones rise as a reward for porn consumption, this is only temporary and can increase the risk of tolerance and dependence on the said behavior. Porn only serves as a distraction from their problems (Coleman, 1987). It is not solving the root cause of their problem, and since addiction will trap the affected person in a loop of unhealthy habits, they may take longer to realize that they are not actually productive.

Chemical dependence. People who have a pertinent history or an ongoing case of substance abuse are at high risk for pornographic addiction (Coleman, 1987). In addition to their tendency to be caught up in another form of addiction, patients who are dependent on any substance of abuse are likely to have a lack of self-discipline and focus to prevent themselves from doing acts which are pleasurable yet detrimental to their health. On top of a lack of self-control, this speaks to the capacity of their brain to function well and think rationally about how to fight the urge to take in pornographic content. Most, if not all, forms of addictive substances have been investigated to affect cognition, such as alcoholic beverages and illicit drugs, which predispose someone to commit high-risk activities, even if that means winding up addicted to another substance or behavior (Vik et al., 2004). It is not uncommon to see people who are addicted to multiple substances and forms of behavior. This emphasizes the vulnerability of people who have a history of addiction, to other forms of addiction, even to pornography.

Changes in behavioral patterns. While this is perceived to have multiple components in the personality of people involved, changes in behavior create patterns that can lead up to pornographic addiction. These behaviors can be psychosexual, compulsive, impulsive, or even addictive in nature (Coleman, 1987). Apart from the original personality the person has in childhood, as they grow up, they may be exposed to various factors that can change their behavior from their inherent personalities. Firstly, they may encounter life-altering events that can change their point of view about matters. People who have lost their loved ones at an early age, or those who may have come from broken families, may unconsciously seek love elsewhere, sometimes even in virtual beings. Next, some people may be exposed to environments that would have to force them to live a non-conventional lifestyle. For example, people who have been coerced to work in prostitution usually encounter any form of addiction to cope with their hostility towards the job and their managers (Roe-Sepowitz et al 2014). There are also some instances where addiction has been inevitably encountered in their work as street-based sex workers, as they may be forced to take in drugs to be less guarded against their clients (El-Bassel et al., 2001). Finally, the culture one grew up in would have a great effect on the personality of the individual. Many people come from a religious group, which may seem more limiting when it comes to sexual expression. This can lead to forced scrupulosity, which serves as a barrier to natural sexual maturity. People cope differently from this. Some have the intense discipline to follow their religious and cultural beliefs, no matter how limiting they are in the natural growth of a person. Some people may give in to their natural urges, but adopt an unorthodox way of expressing sexuality secretly. Because these people are told that sexual expression is against their beliefs, they may resort to discreet ways of sexual expressions, such as consuming pornography for self-gratification, masturbating to digital sexual content, and searching for more sexual content on the web to gain experiences they can't have in real life.

Epidemiology

Pornographic addiction has rapidly increased as a result of the ease of availability of Internet use. While seeing naked people may not be problematic with one look, the various cocktail of pleasure hormones that it induces in the brain results in compulsion. This leads the person to do it again and again, starting the seemingly endless cycle of addiction. Based on a review, compulsive sexual behavior includes pornography consumption, as well as self-gratification, sexual encounters with strangers, exploring infidelity, fetishistic behaviors, and even prostitution (Coleman, 1987). Sexual activities can branch off to other activities, in the spirit of exploration, curiosity, and pleasure.

The risk of being addicted to pornography is calculated due to the presence of the "Triple A" influence comprising the triad of **accessibility, affordability,** and **anonymity,** as described by Cooper's (1998). Three factors are elaborated as follows: Accessibility, due to the mostly unregulated use of web; affordability, due to the widespread availability of the Internet with even the developing countries catching up to the tech wave; and anonymity, encouraging people to consume strongly sexual content, without the corresponding consequences. This three-factor explanation makes pornographic content wildly viral nowadays (De Alarcón et al., 2019).

Various people are at risk for addiction due to pornographic exposure. The main people at risk for comorbidity of having pornographic addiction are the youth who are vulnerable to addictive habits without the benefit of a mature mind (De Alarcón et al., 2019). In the long run, this may affect the proper sexual maturity, development, and overall productive function in the youth.

While pornography consumption and addiction are well-known concepts, these remain difficult to objectively assess. In light of this, various research instruments have been developed to assess pornographic addiction as objectively as possible, while overcoming such limitations (Cacioppo et al., 2018).

- Cyber-Pornography Use Inventory (Grubbs et al., 2010)
- Compulsive Pornography Compulsion (Noor et al., 2014)
- Hypersexual Behavior Inventory (Reid et al., 2011)
- Compulsive Sexual Behavior Inventory (Coleman et al., 2001)
- Sexual Addiction Screening Test-Revised (Carnes et al., 2010)
- Internet Sex Screening Test (Delmonico and Miller, 2003)
- Inventory of Problematic Online Experiences (Mitchell et al., 2009)
- Pornography Consumption Inventory (Reid et al., 2010)

Pornographic addiction remains to present some difficulty in terms of objective assessment. Such challenges are due to some research limitations including sampling bias, lack of appropriate diagnostic instrumentals, opposing approximations to the concept, and the possibility of overlapping pathology with other conditions (i.e., sex addiction) that may be related to or are parallel to their symptomatology. Nevertheless, it is a topic that must be studied well because of the growing number of Internet users who may be exposed to pornography and may be at risk for addiction.

The pathophysiology of addiction to pornography

The core of porn addiction is its capacity to embed itself in the regular habits of an individual. Without it, it would be like watching a movie once and mostly not watching it again because you already know what's in it. With habit formation, consuming pornography does not only entail the act of watching but also being mindful of the arousing stimulus, acting on it, and obtaining an unearned pleasure as a reward. This keeps the person coming back again, seeking pornographic content for a highly accessible source of sexual gratification.

Establishing the habit loop. The core of addiction is a solid habit loop (Chen et al., 2020). Taking advantage of the pleasure as a reward that is gained from every pornographic viewing session, porn consumption is easily formed into a habit with an almost omnipresent stimulus of anything arousing to the person and with a reward of dopamine boost for instant pleasure. With long-term use of pornography, the mind can undergo neuroplasticity and rewire its regions to best suit a brain overdosed on dopamine (Hilton, 2013).

Stimuli. Like any physiologic response, habits start with a stimulus (Chen, 2020). Sexual stimulation is usually induced by multisensory stimuli and imaginative experiences to mimic impending sexual activity. These include feelings of erotic touch on the erogenous zones, the scent of a potential mate, and the appreciation of flattering secondary characteristics, in addition to the imagination of sexual stimuli. While this is natural in actual sex, pornographic consumption does not have the scent aspect of the stimuli, and self-induced tactile stimuli are meant to stimulate the person himself. Digital pornographic content limits stimuli to the sight of flesh from nude actors, sexually suggestive photos, and the act of sexual intercourse as seen on the screen. This allows the individual to be aroused just by photos on their computer screens.

Action. The activity itself undertaken by a person forming habits is the action (Chen, 2020). The action accompanying porn consumption usually involves self-gratification. While there are no limits to what one can do to act on their stimuli, masturbation is one of the most common actions correlated with porn consumption. Masturbation is one of the primitive ways of self-gratification, but when made into a habit, it wreaks havoc on the neurochemical balance of the brain. When the time comes when tolerance to porn and masturbation kicks in, curiosity will fuel these affected people to explore other activities such as mutual masturbation, voyeurism, sadism, sexual intercourse with a stranger, fetishism, and even non-consensual sexual activities. These will be done for the sake of the release of pleasure hormones and will imprint other activities to induce dopamine release from stimuli that are not supposed to elicit it.

Reward. The reward is one of the most important parts of porn addiction. Regardless of the actions undertaken by the affected individual in the action phase, the temporary pleasure at the end is usually the motivation to push through with this activity (Chen, 2020). Despite the hype on how pleasure can be a positive experience, it takes too much energy and time to achieve a few seconds of satisfaction. Moreover, chronic self-induction of dopamine boosts is not sustainable as it may lead to tolerance and dependence, similar to other forms of addiction. When this happens, it would take much greater effort to achieve the very same level of reward.

Adopting pleasure-seeking habits

After the habit loop is established, the anticipated effects can be expected as well (Chen, 2020). After all, it's not only the affected people who have this urge. The difference between the sexual urges of normal people and those who are addicted to pornography is the motivation to get into an activity to act on the urge—normal people would have their rational minds intact during sexual urges, and thus will know when and when not to act on it, while the addicted person will have no self-control, discipline, and motivation to fight their urges. This will result in certain consequences when porn consumption results in a grave loss in productivity in the long run.

High dopamine rush. While we get dopamine rush in various things that we find pleasurable, self-inducing it is not sustainable and can lead to addiction. In acute to sub-acute utilization of self-induced pleasure, the dopamine boost accompanying the reward will take a toll on the imbalance of the neurochemistry of the brain. This will use up dopamine reserves for other normal functions, such as emotional regulation, cognitive function, and other neurophysiologic functions. In chronic utilization of self-gratification, dopamine high would be harder to reach, due to developing tolerance, which means that it would take more intensive degrees of action, such as porn consumption and sexual activity, to attain the sexual satisfaction one used to have before they were addicted (Hilton, 2013).

Consequences apparent in the long run. Chronic use of pleasure-inducing activity can lead to addiction, which by extension, has its own consequences. It can alter one's whole personality, the behavior that usually defines them, and their overall health and wellness. For example, addiction to pornography can lead to other conditions that are overtly sexual in nature. A similar condition that may be a significant comorbidity of pornography addiction is hypersexual disorder (De Alarcón et al., 2019). This may lead to other high-risk sexual activities that can worsen their condition. Their general health and well-being will be affected as well, as imbalances in neurotransmitters may lead to disequilibrium in cognitive and mental functions. This makes people addicted to pornography and any other sexual activities prone to mental disorders such as depressive disorder, anxiety disorder, and even stress disorders. Personality can also be affected as constant exposure to pornography can alter one's personality and behavior. Some people may end up with antisocial personalities, being highly dependent on digital pornographic materials to get by their day, while others may develop narcissistic and histrionic personalities, as they embody their idols in the adult entertainment industry.

Making time and taking time. While it is challenging to study this condition, porn addiction, along with other behavioral addictions comprise the same set of pathogenesis: lack of self-control, high-risk utilization of the material, and overall impairment (De Alarcón et al., 2019). This can eventually impair their personal, social, and professional lives, as the habit of pornographic consumption requires time, and energy. The time that should have been allotted for a meaningful Friday night with close school friends can turn into a night in solitary watching of their newly downloaded pornographic videos. The energy that should have been allotted for meeting people who could be one's potential partner can turn into a cybersex session with strangers online. The mind of an addict is oriented to make time and allot energy for pornographic consumption within their day, making it a regular affair, which strongly predisposes them to long-term porn use and eventually, addiction.

Recovery from porn addiction and its challenges

In people attempting to recover, they may encounter challenges as well. Tolerance, dependence, and withdrawal are some of the most pressing challenges of behavioral addiction, including chronic pornography use. Another emerging problem in general addiction withdrawal syndromes is when individuals attempting to recover from substance addictions seek other replacement mechanisms, such as porn addiction (Tadpatrikar & Sharma, 2018). In an effort to curb down use of addicting substances, such as illicit drugs, sugar, or alcohol, the brain naturally seeks other sources of dopamine, to sustain the losses by abstinence to the substance. This puts recovering addicts at risk for relapse or for a new set of addiction, they would find in porn consumption. On top of this, sexual gratification using porn is a powerful source of instant dopamine rush and can effectively sustain the addictive mechanism that is lost from the withdrawal.

Over the past 10 years or so, I have helped hundreds of people who have fallen into this endless cycle—and one of the best treatment methods I have implemented is what is known as the Critical Alignment Model Recovery Program. The program relies heavily on monitoring, modifying and improving four critical areas, which are:

1. Environment
2. Structure or system
3. Implementing strategies
4. People in your circle.

Environment:

Environment breeds actions. Unless you clean up your current environment to become conducive to productive work, faith-driven activities, good habits etc., you will keep on falling back to your compulsive habits.

Your environment usually consists of places that you often visit, people that you always meet and interact with, and objects that you usually use or see. Whatever the case is, you must secure these places, filter those people, especially those who have negative impacts on your behaviors, and get rid of any objects or item that maybe is a trigger for your porn consumption. And if you cannot eliminate these objects completely, such as your cell phones or computer devices, then at least protect them using blockers and other software to ensure that you are safe from accessing these images.

Structure/System:

You cannot live without a structure in life, a system that governs all your behaviors. Dos and don'ts, decisions about executing different and healthier habits, jotting down a complete list of actions to practice immediately, actions to practice in the future, and actions that you shouldn't participate in at all.

Bear in mind that what makes this step work very well is making it public. You must tell people around you about that system, because even though you might feel resisted by their judgmental remarks sometimes, in the long run, they will be the ones to assist you to apply your own structure because they have sensed that you are dead serious about it.

Implementation:

This is the hardest part, because it requires a mind-shift and deep belief within yourself that you can get things done.

So how can you achieve this?

- Keep your eye on the WHY. You must draft down your vision in life. Why is it so important for you to quit porn? If your reason is not big enough, you might not develop the necessary energy to fight this monster.
- Ignore the pain associated with good actions. Any good (or even bad) action requires effort. And exerting effort is not always a pleasant experience. But it is pushing one's limit against this annoyance that gets the job done. So don't let any sort of pain stop you from keeping the momentum of recovery up.

People:

If we said that implementation is the hardest part in recovery, involving people is the one step that usually scares addicts the most. But the sad news (for them) is, that without a support system from people who love you the most, there's no chance for you to fight addiction on your own. So you have to take this step as quickly as you can. Perhaps you can start by getting in touch with people online first, using platforms like Reboot Nation or NoFap communities. But I always encourage those who are addicted to porn to find REAL people in their circle to assist them on a regular basis by monitoring their devices, checking on their schedule, listening to their struggles, dragging them out of their bedrooms into nature and so on.

Without these 4 elements in place, recovery will always seem impossible.

References:

[1] Brown, C. C., Durtschi, J. A., Carroll, J. S., & Willoughby, B. J. (2017). Understanding and predicting classes of college students who use pornography. Computers in Human Behavior, 66, 114-121.

[2] Kort, J. (2015). Pornography, addiction to ("pro"). The International Encyclopedia of Human Sexuality, 861–1042. doi:10.1002/9781118896877.wbiehs360

[3] Olose, E. O., Busari, C. O., Anake, G. A., Adubina, B. I., & Ogundare, T. (2021). Pornography Addiction in a University Undergraduate: a Case Report. World Journal of Medical Sciences, 18(2), 97-102.

Tadpatrikar, A., & Sharma, M. K. (2018). Pornography as a replacement for substance use: An emerging approach to understand addiction mechanism. Open Journal of Psychiatry & Allied Sciences, 9(2), 173-175.

De Alarcón, R., de la Iglesia, J., Casado, N., & Montejo, A. (2019). Online Porn Addiction: What We Know and What We Don't—A Systematic Review. Journal of Clinical Medicine, 8(1), 91. doi:10.3390/jcm8010091

Pyle, T. M., & Bridges, A. J. (2012). Perceptions of relationship satisfaction and addictive behavior: Comparing pornography and marijuana use. Journal of Behavioral Addictions, 1(4), 171–179. doi:10.1556/jba.1.2012.007

Cacioppo, M., Gori, A., Schimmenti, A., Baiocco, R., Laghi, F., & Caretti, V. (2018). Development of a new screening tool for cyber pornography: Psychometric properties of the Cyber Pornography Addiction Test (CYPAT). Clinical neuropsychiatry, 15(1).

World Health Organization. (2019). ICD-11: International classification of diseases 11th revision.

American Psychiatric Association (2022). Diagnostic and statistical manual of mental disorders (5th ed., text rev.). https://doi.org/10.1176/appi.books.9780890425787

Vik, P. W., Cellucci, T., Jarchow, A., & Hedt, J. (2004). Cognitive impairment in substance abuse. Psychiatric Clinics, 27(1), 97–109.

Roe-Sepowitz, D. E., Gallagher, J., Hickle, K. E., Pérez Loubert, M., & Tutelman, J. (2014). Project ROSE: An Arrest Alternative for Victims of Sex Trafficking and Prostitution. Journal of Offender Rehabilitation, 53(1), 57–74. doi:10.1080/10509674.2013.861323

El-Bassel, N., Witte, S. S., Wada, T., Gilbert, L., & Wallace, J. (2001). Correlates of Partner Violence Among Female Street-Based Sex Workers: Substance Abuse, History of Childhood Abuse, and HIV Risks. AIDS Patient Care and STDs, 15(1), 41–51. doi:10.1089/108729101460092

Grubbs, J. B., Sessoms, J., Wheeler, D. M., & Volk, F. (2010). The CyberPornography Use Inventory: The development of a new assessment instrument. Sexual Addiction & Compulsivity 17, 106-126.

Noor, S. W., Rosser, B. S., & Erickson, D.J (2014). A brief scale to measure problematic sexually explicit media consumption: Psychometric properties of the Compulsive Pornography Consumption (CPC) scale among men who have sex with men. Sexual Addiction & Compulsivity 21, 3, 240-261

Reid, R. C., Garos, S., & Carpenter, B. N. (2011). Reliability, validity, and psychometric development of the hypersexual behaviour inventory in an outpatient sample of men. Sexual Addiction & Compulsivity 18, 1, 30-51.

Coleman, E., Miner, M., Ohlerking, F., & Raymond, N. (2001). Compulsive Sexual Behavior Inventory: A preliminary study of reliability and validity. Journal of Sex and Marital Therapy 27, 325-332

Carnes, P., Green, B., & Carnes, S. (2010). The same yet different: Refocusing the sexual addiction screening test (SAST) to reflect orientation and gender. Sexual Addiction & Compulsivity 17, 1, 7-30.

Delmonico, D. L., & Miller, J. A. (2003). The internet sex screening test: A comparison of sexual compulsives versus non-sexual compulsives. Sexual and Relationship Therapy 18, 261-276.

Mitchell, K. J., Sabina, C., Finkelhor, D., & Wells, M. (2009). Index of problematic online experiences: Item characteristics and correlation with negative symptomatology. Cyberpsychology & Behavior 12, 6, 707-711.

Hilton, D. L. (2013). Pornography addiction – a supranormal stimulus considered in the context of neuroplasticity. Socioaffective Neuroscience & Psychology, 3(1), 20767. doi:10.3402/snp.v3i0.20767

Chen, W., Chan, T. W., Wong, L. H., Looi, C. K., Liao, C. C. Y., Cheng, H. N. H., ... Pi, Z. (2020). IDC theory: habit and the habit loop. Research and Practice in Technology Enhanced Learning, 15(1). doi:10.1186/s41039-020-00127-7

Chen, W., Chan, T. W., Wong, L. H., Looi, C. K., Liao, C. C. Y., Cheng, H. N. H., ... Pi, Z. (2020). IDC theory: habit and the habit loop. Research and Practice in Technology Enhanced Learning, 15(1). doi:10.1186/s41039-020-00127-7

Duffy, A., Dawson, D. L., & das Nair, R. (2016). Pornography Addiction in Adults: A Systematic Review of Definitions and Reported Impact. The Journal of Sexual Medicine, 13(5), 760–777. doi:10.1016/j.jsxm.2016.03.002

FINAL WORD

The main intention of this book was to call to action all mental health professionals, psychologists, psychiatrists, and medical experts to approach the issue of widespread porn consumption with a critical lens, by recognizing the addictive characteristics of pornography and the detrimental effects it can have on individuals. Only then, we can work towards a lasting solution for those who have been badly impacted.

I know that the DSM-5, the most recent edition of the Diagnostic and Statistical Manual of Mental Disorders, did not include a diagnosis for pornography addiction. However, this does not mean that we should ignore the thousands of people around the world who do experience problematic compulsive behaviors related to pornography consumption. As I have demonstrated throughout the book, mental health professionals and researchers are already using the term "pornography addiction" to describe the patterns of behaviors that resemble drug addiction, such as difficulty controlling the behavior, negative consequences in relationships, work or studies, and even withdrawal symptoms when attempting to quit. So, it would be irresponsible to look at those who are suffering day and night due to their addiction to pornography and act as if nothing is wrong with them or with porn in general.

The evidence supporting the reality of the harms induced by pornographic exposure is crystal clear, as the impacts are very damaging and mentally draining. Such exposure can diminish our capacity for productivity and sap our energy, as well as potentially affect the fundamental and physical structure of our brains, resulting in a variety of severe mental illnesses and disorders, which require the immediate intervention of specialists.

Failure to address this challenge in a timely manner may have catastrophic implications, as the looming presence of this issue threatens to consume us all.

For those who wish to reach out to the Aware Academy for assistance, you can send us an email at info@awareacademy.com.au

All the best.
Wael Ibrahim

NOTES

Notes

_____

_____

_____

_____

_____

_____

_____

_____

_____

_____

_____

_____

_____

_____

Notes

www.ingramcontent.com/pod-product-compliance
Lightning Source LLC
Chambersburg PA
CBHW022052020426
42335CB00012B/654